PRACTICAL MICROBIOLOGY
for
DENTAL STUDENTS

RELATED BOOKS OF INTEREST

Textbook of Microbiology, 3rd ed. .... D.R. Arora / B. Arora
Medical Parasitology, 2nd ed. .... D.R. Arora / B. Arora
Textbook of Microbiology for Dental Students, 2nd ed. .... D.R. Arora / Hina Arora
Microbiology for Nurses and Allied Sciences .... D.R. Arora / B. Arora
Practical Microbiology .... Bharti Arora / D.R. Arora

PRACTICAL MICROBIOLOGY
for
DENTAL STUDENTS

Bharti Arora M.D.
Assistant Professor, Department of Microbiology,
Maharaja Agrasen Medical College,
Agroha, Hisar, Haryana (India)

D.R. Arora M.D., Ph.D., M.N.A.M.S.
Professor & Head, Department of Microbiology,
Maharaja Agarsen Medical College, Agroha, Hisar, Haryana (India)
Lead Assessor, Faculty Member and Member Technical Committee,
National Accreditation Board for Testing and Calibration Laboratories (NABL),
New Delhi (India)
Assessor, National Accreditation Board for Hospitals and Healthcare Providers (NABH),
New Delhi (India)
Formerly Professor & Head, Department of Microbiology,
Postgraduate Institute of Medical Sciences, Rohtak, Haryana (India)
Ex W.H.O. Fellow; and Visiting Professor, University of Mauritius

CBS

CBS PUBLISHERS & DISTRIBUTORS PVT. LTD.
NEW DELHI • BANGALORE • PUNE • COCHIN • CHENNAI (INDIA)

ISBN : 978-81-239-1595-1

First Edition : 2008
Reprint : 2012

Published by Satish Kumar Jain and produced by V.K. Jain for
CBS Publishers & Distributors Pvt. Ltd.,
CBS Plaza, 4819/XI Prahlad Street, 24 Ansari Road, Daryaganj,
New Delhi - 110002, India. • Website: www.cbspd.com
e-mail: delhi@cbspd.com, cbspubs@airtelmail.in
Ph.: 23289259, 23266861, 23266867 • Fax: 011-23243014

Branches:

- ***Bengaluru:*** Seema House, 2975, 17th Cross, K.R. Road,
  Bansankari 2nd Stage, Bengaluru - 560070 Ph.: +91-80-26771678/79
  • E-mail: cbsbng@gmail.com, bangalore@cbspd.com
- ***Pune:*** Bhuruk Prestige, Sr. No. 52/12/2+1+3/2,
  Narhe, Haveli (Near Katraj-Dehu Road By-pass), Pune - 411051
  Ph.: +91-20-64704058/59, 32342277 • E-mail: pune@cbspd.com
- ***Kochi:*** 36/14, Kalluvilakam, Lissie Hospital Road,
  Kochi - 682018, Kerala • Ph.: +91-484-4059061-65
  Fax: +91-484-4059065 • E-mail: cochin@cbspd.com
- ***Chennai:*** 20, West Park Road, Shenoy Nagar, Chennai - 600030
  Ph.: +91-44-26260666, 26208620 E-mail: chennai@cbspd.com

Printed at :
India Binding House, Noida (UP)

Preface

For qualifying an examination a microbiology student has to get through in theory and practical separately. Though a large number of theory books in microbiology are available, no good book covering practical aspects is available. Keeping in view the above, a simple and comprehensive book on practical aspects of all sections of microbiology has been devised. This book has been divided into nine parts that include general bacteriology, serology/immunology, parasitology, systemic bacteriology, mycology, virology, recent advances, spots and appendices. Each practical exercise ends with important questions and their answers which help the student to prepare for theory, practical and viva voce examination.

This book is meant for BDS, BSc MLT, MSc, MSC MLT students and technical staff of medical (clinical) laboratories. It is a 'bench book' containing well tried methods. This will also help the students preparing for postgraduate entrance examination.

We express our sincere thanks to Dr. Amit Arora for proof-reading, invaluable suggestions and continuous encouragement. We are deeply indebted to Dr. (Mrs.) B. Arora, Professor and Head, Department of Pathology, Postgraduate Institute of Medical Sciences, Rohtak, for contributing photomicrographs and valuable suggestions. We owe our debt of gratitude to Dr. Harender and Mr. Prabhat Ranjan for proof-reading and for meticulously drawing all the figures. Thanks are also due to Mr. Dharamvir, Mr. Kuldeep and Mr. Parveen Sharma for composing this book, Mr. B.R. Sharma for encouragement and M/s CBS Publishers & Distributors for their cooperation and keen interest in the publication of this book.

Bharti Arora
D.R. Arora

Instructions

General Instructions to the Students for Safety

- Protect your clothings in the laboratory by wearing an overall. This should not be worn outside the laboratory.
- All microorganisms should be regarded as capable of causing disease.
- Long hair should be tied back to avoid risks from fire and accidental contamination.
- Mouth-pipetting should not be done.
- Always flame the bacteriological loop before and after use.
- Do not try to smell any bacterial culture.
- Do not expose microbiological cultures longer than necessary.
- Do not shake liquid cultures.
- Do not place cotton-wool plugs or other stoppers on the bench.
- Do not place contaminated pipettes on the bench top.
- Do not sit on the bench top.
- Do not lick labels with tongue.
- Do not put pencils, fingers and other objects in your mouth.
- Do not eat or drink in the laboratory.
- Discard the used and contaminated slides and other material in disinfectant jar.
- Do not wander about in the laboratory.
- Do not forcibly expel material from a pipette.
- Always wash your hands thoroughly at the end of your work.
- Bench tops should be disinfected immediately after experiment is over.
- All accidents like cuts and burns in the laboratory should be reported to your teacher.
- Accidental spillage of bacterial growth or other contaminated material should be reported to your teacher or laboratory technician.

PLATE I

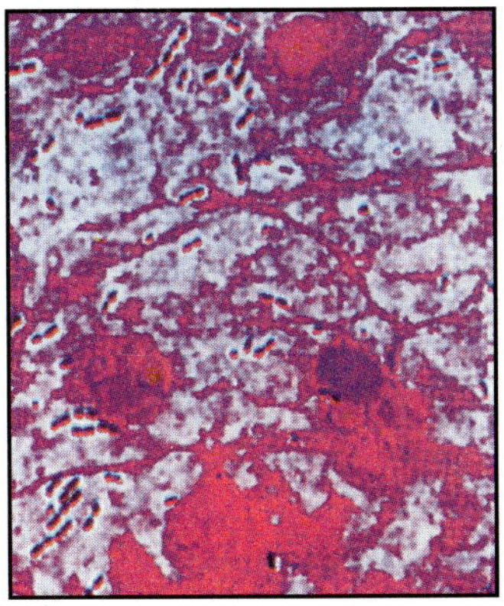

Fig. 1. Gram-stained smear showing Gram-positive diplococci.

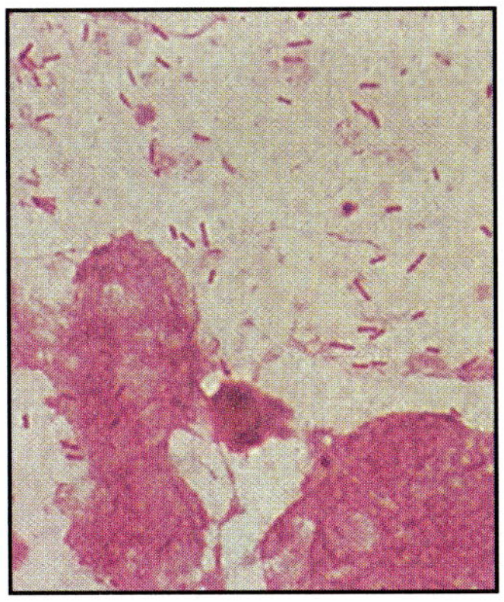

Fig. 2. Gram-stained smear showing Gram-negative bacilli.

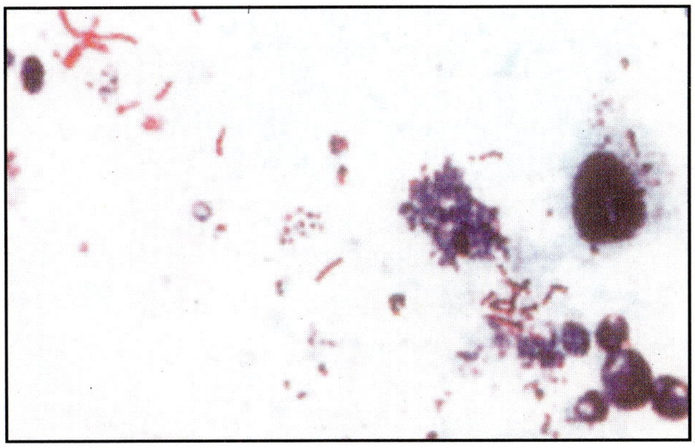

Fig. 3. Sputum smear showing acid-fast bacilli.

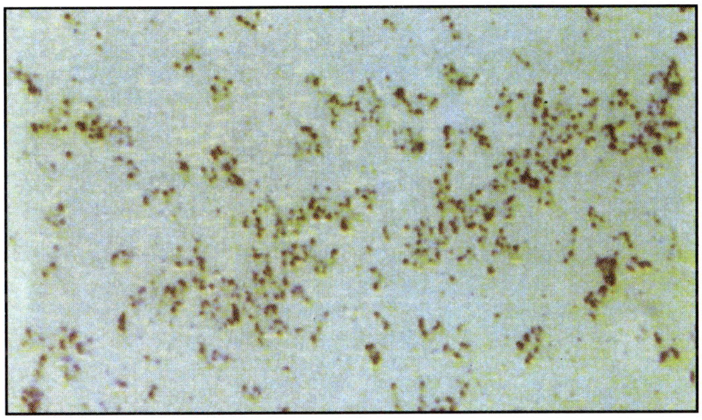

Fig. 4. *Corynebacterium diphtheriae* showing metachromatic granules.

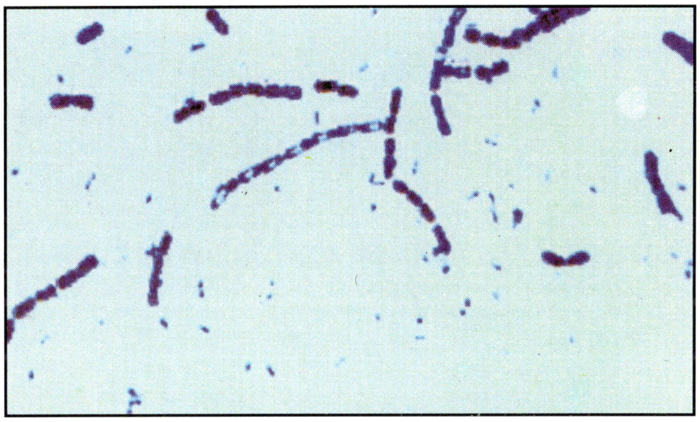

Fig. 5. Gram-stained smear of *Bacillus subtilis* showing Gram-positive bacilli in chains with spores which appear as unstained areas within the bacilli.

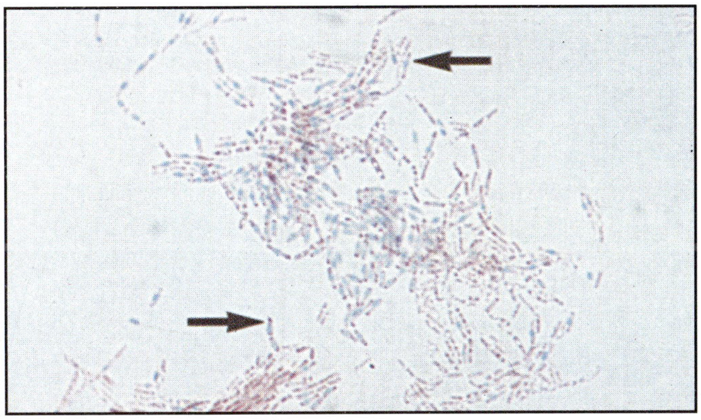

Fig. 6. Malachite green stained smear of *Bacillus cereus* showing red bacilli with green spores.

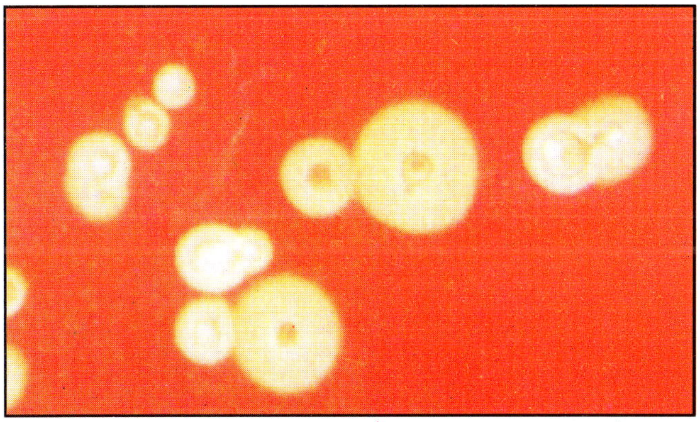

Fig. 7. An India ink wet mount of *Cryptococcus neoformans* showing encapsulated budding yeast cells.

PLATE II

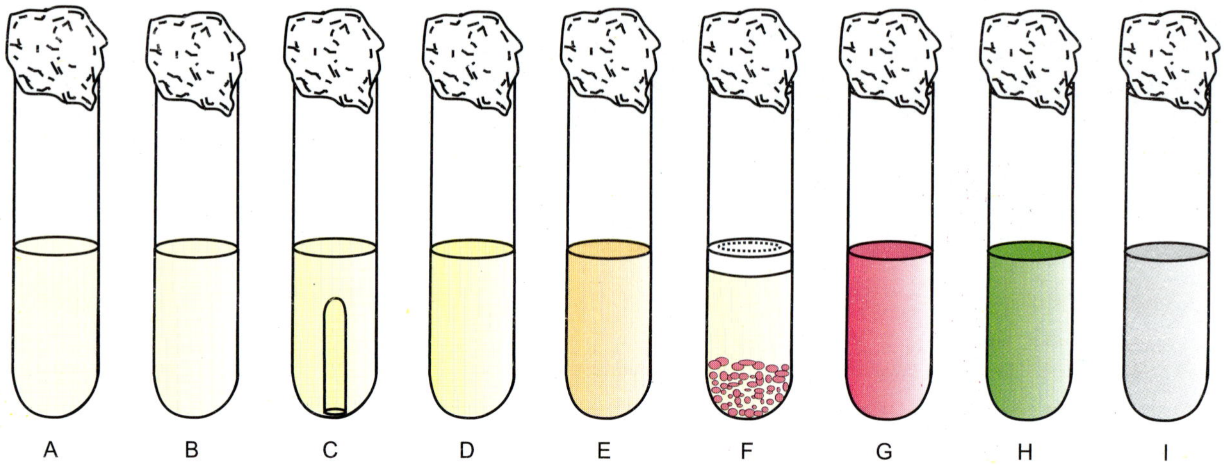

Fig. 8. (A) Peptone water, (B) Nutrient broth, (C) Sugar medium, (D) Glucose broth, (E) Bile broth, (F) Cooked meat broth, (G) Buffered glycerol saline, (H) Brilliant green tetrathionate broth, and (I) Selenite F broth.

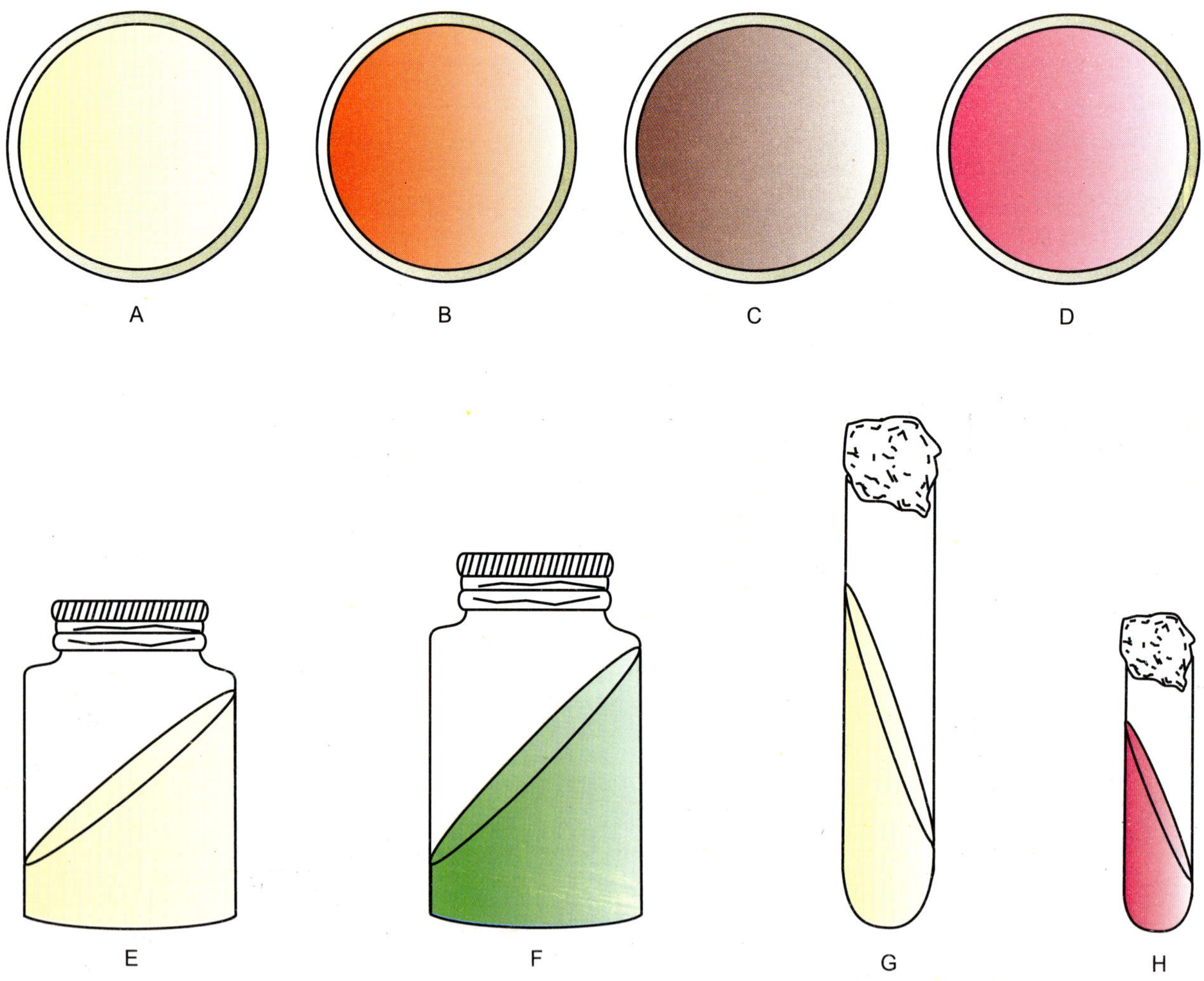

Fig. 9. (A) Nutrient agar, (B) Blood agar, (C) Chocolate agar, (D) MacConkey agar, (E) Loeffler's serum slope, (F) Lowenstein-Jensen medium, (G) Sabouraud's dextrose agar, and (H) Triple sugar iron agar.

PLATE III

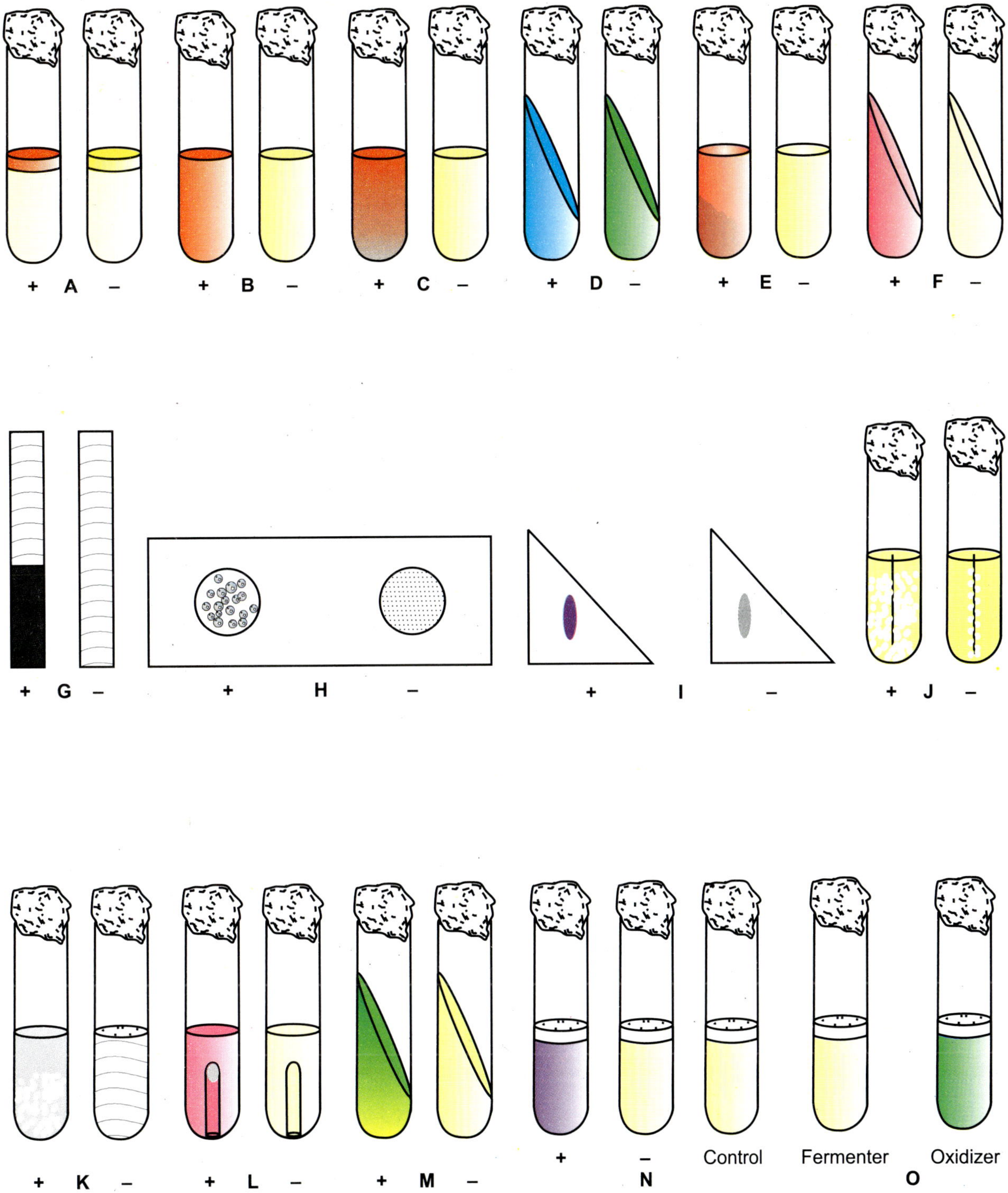

Fig. 10. (A) Indole test, (B) MR test, (C) VP test, (D) Citrate utilization test, (E) Nitrate reduction test, (F) Urease test, (G) H_2S test, (H) Catalase test, (I) Oxidase test, (J) Motility test, (K) Potassium cyanide test, (L) Sugar fermentation test, (M) PPA test, (N) Decarboxylase test, and (O) OF test.

PLATE IV

Eggs, Trophozoites, Cysts and Oocysts in the Stool of Man

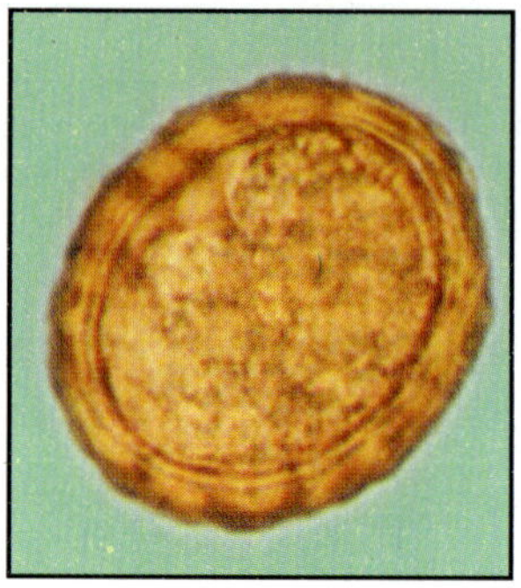

Fig. 11. Fertilized egg of *Ascaris lumbricoides.*

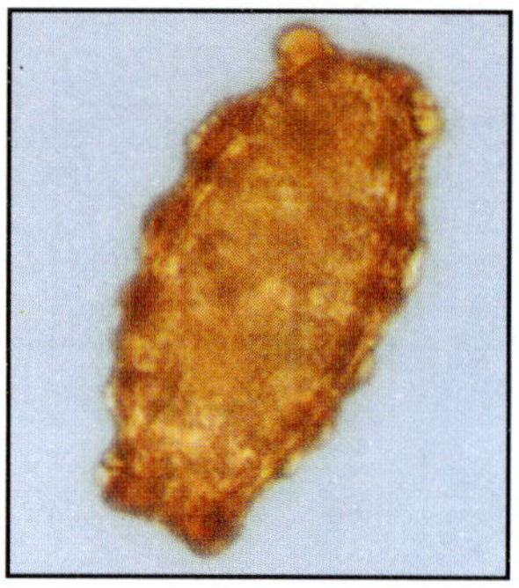

Fig. 12. Unfertilized egg of *Ascaris lumbricoides.*

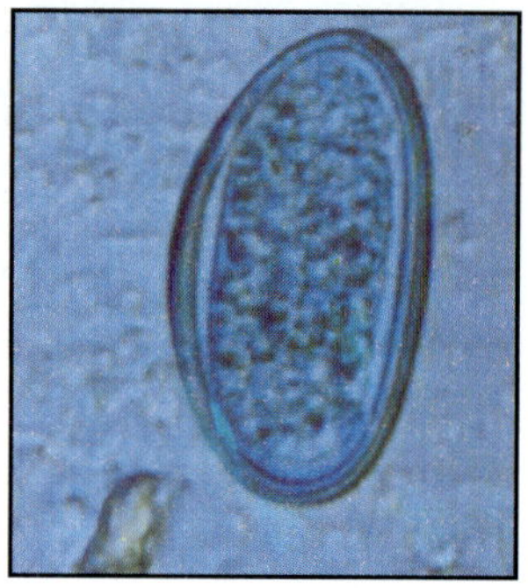

Fig. 13. *Enterobius vermicularis.*

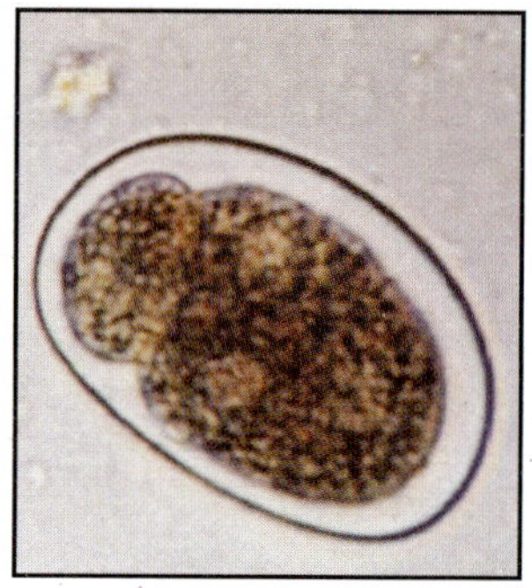

Fig. 14. *Ancylostoma duodenale.*

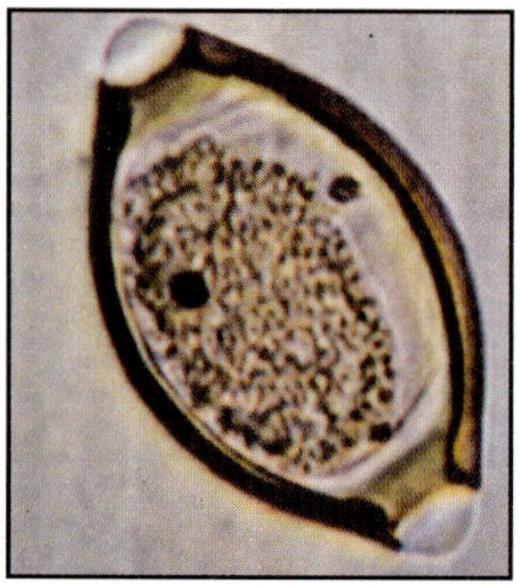

Fig. 15. *Trichuris trichiura.*

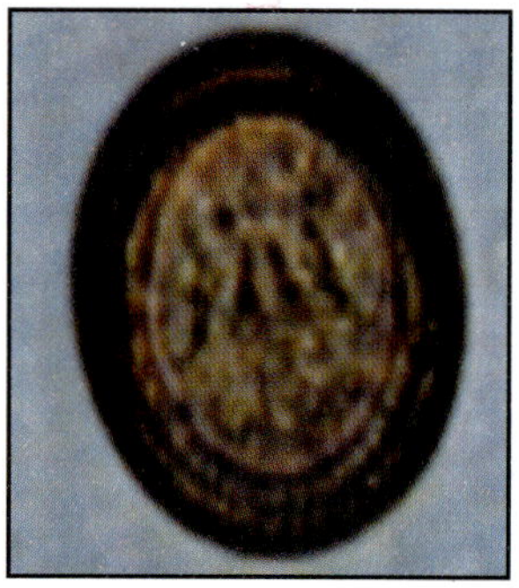

Fig. 16. *Taenia.*

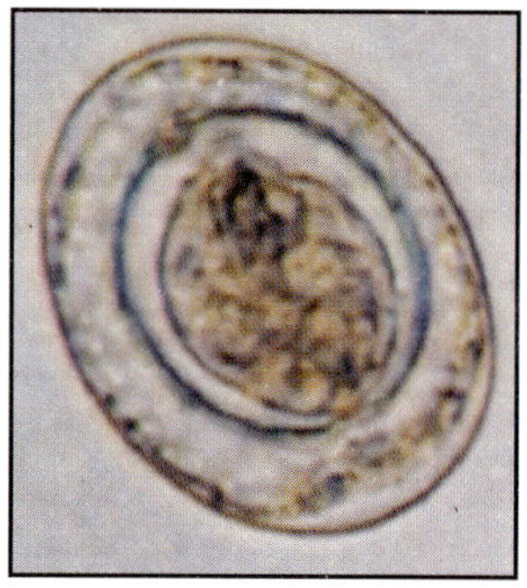

Fig. 17. *Hymenolepis nana.*

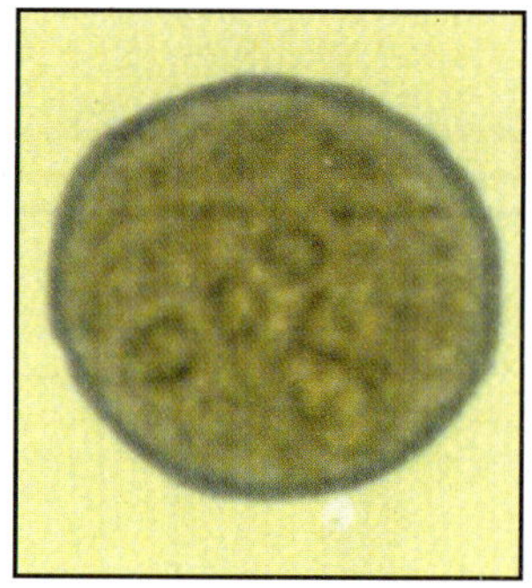

Fig. 18. Cyst of *Entamoeba histolytica* in stool.

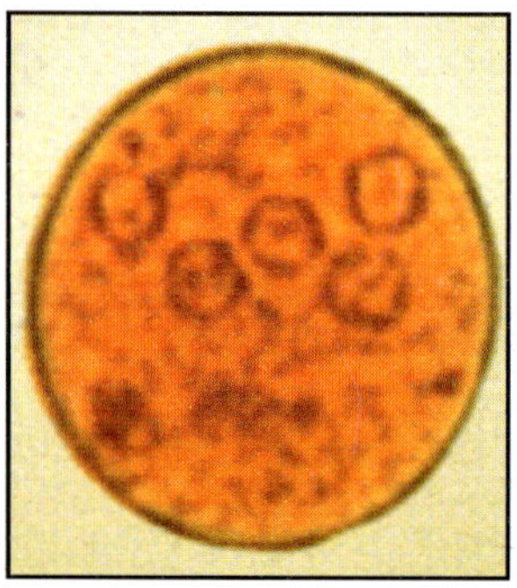

Fig. 19. Cyst of *Entamoeba coli* in stool.

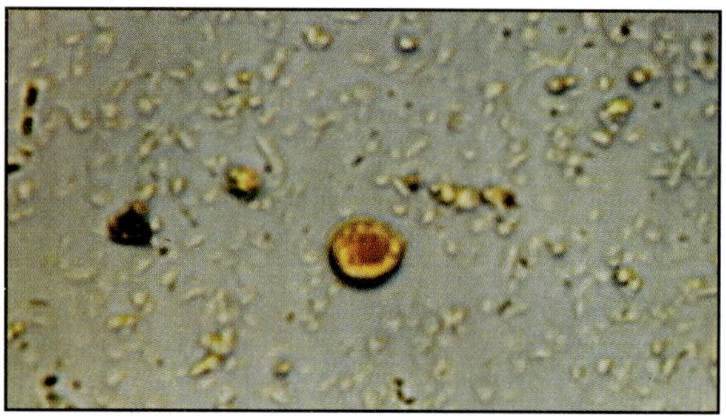

Fig. 20. Cyst of *Iodamoeba buetschlii* in stool.

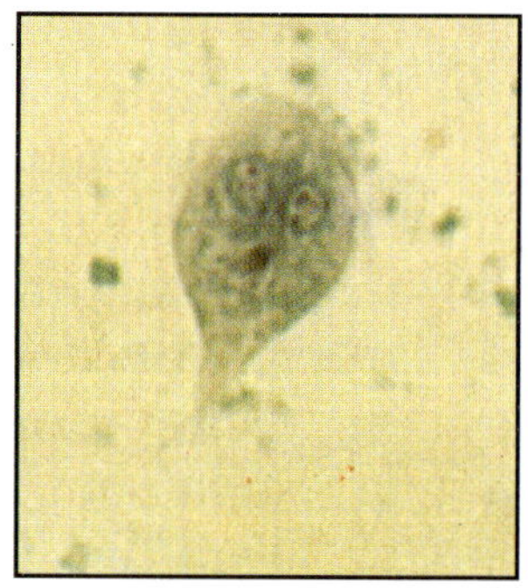

Fig. 21. Trophozoite of *Giardia lamblia* in stool.

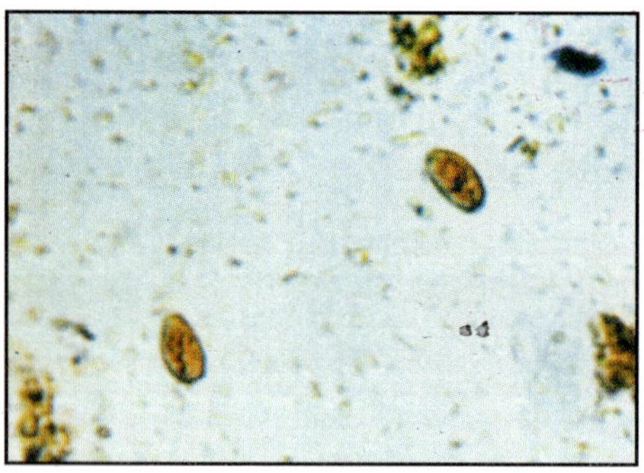

Fig. 22. Cysts of *Giardia lamblia* in stool.

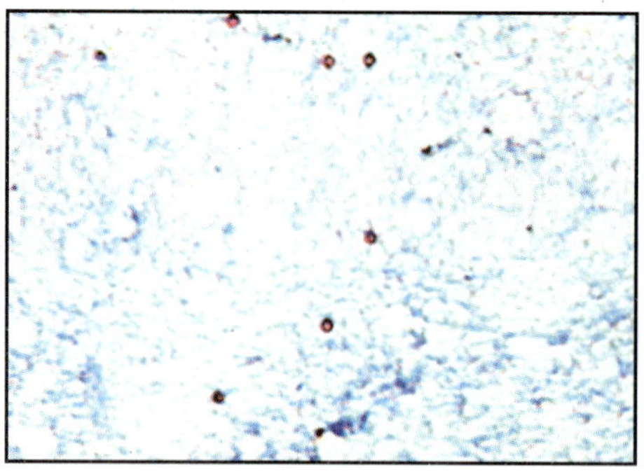

Fig. 23. Oocysts of *Cryptosporidium parvum* in faecal smear stained with modified acid-fast stain.

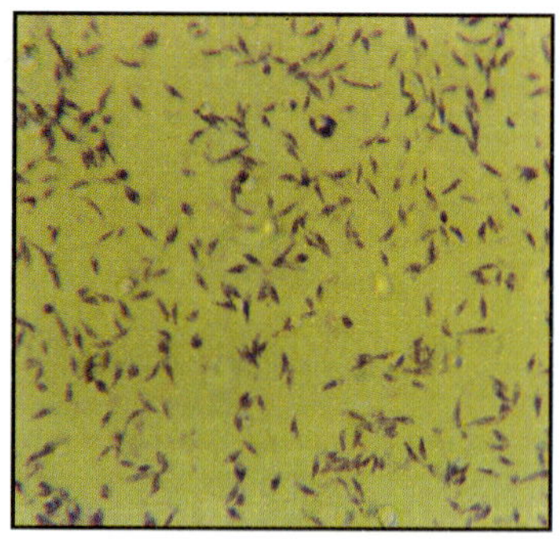

Fig. 24. Promastigote forms of *Leishmania donovani* in culture.

PLATE V

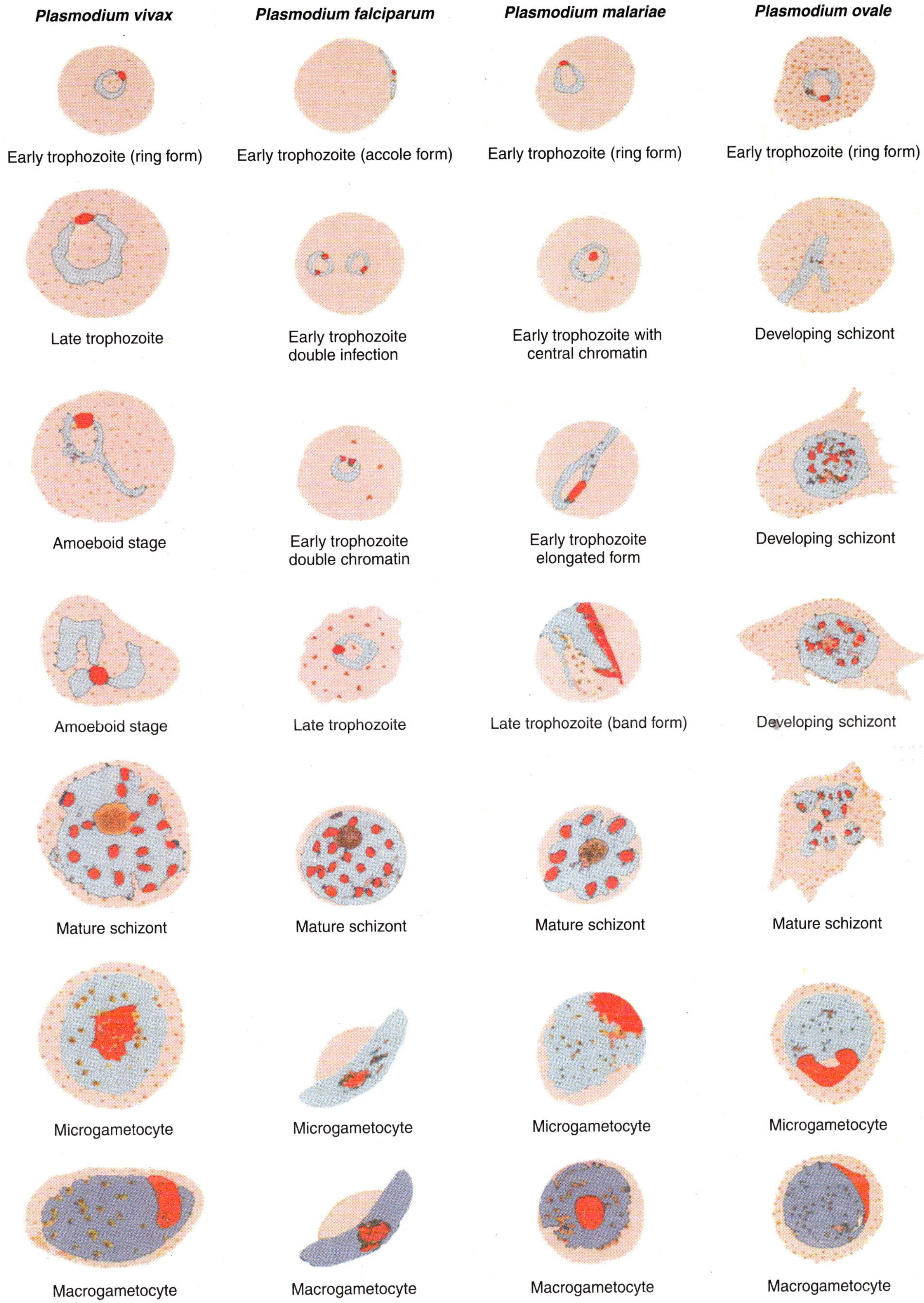

Fig. 25. Morphological forms of malaria parasites.

PLATE VI

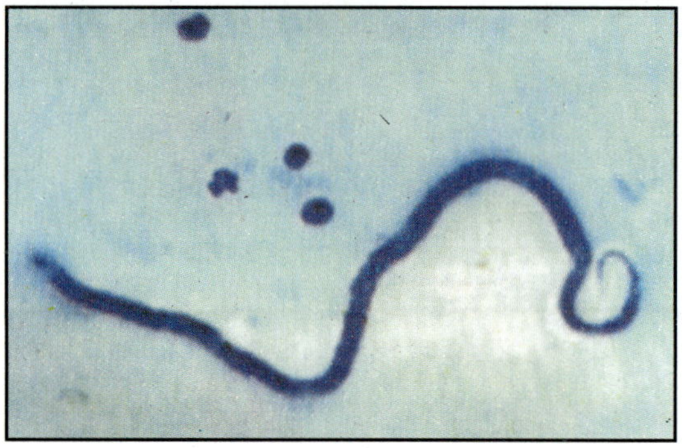

Fig. 26. *Microfilaria bancrofti* in peripheral blood.

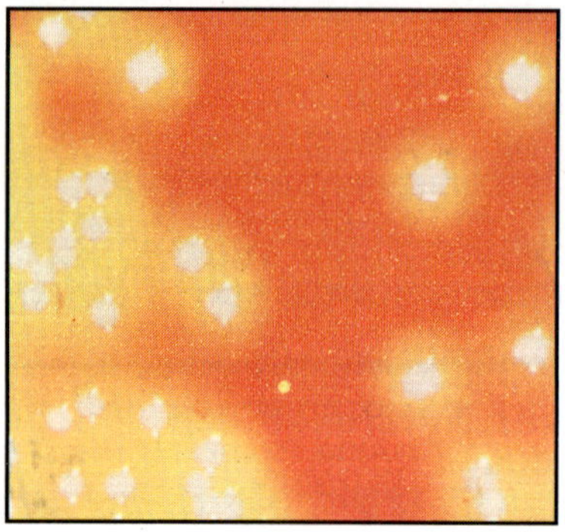

Fig. 27. *Staphylococcus aureus* on blood agar showing β-haemolysis.

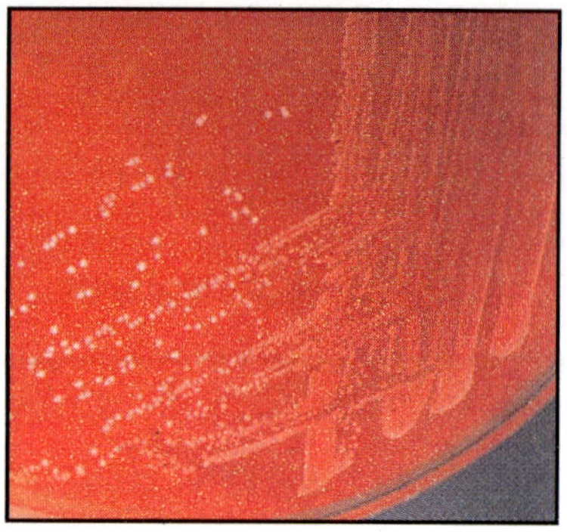

Fig. 28. Coagulase-negative staphylococci growing on blood agar.

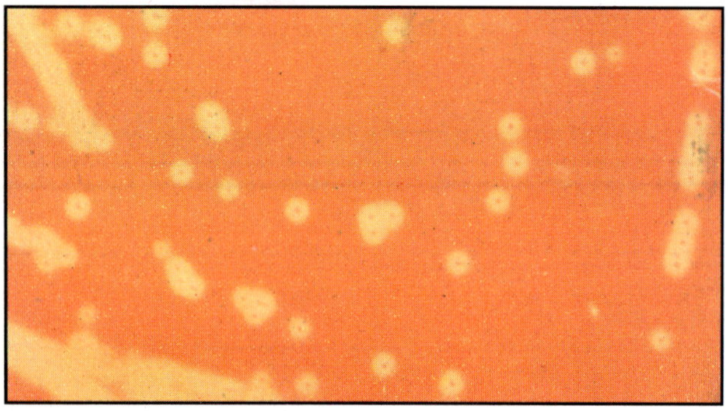

Fig. 29. *Streptococcus pyogenes* on blood agar showing β-haemolysis.

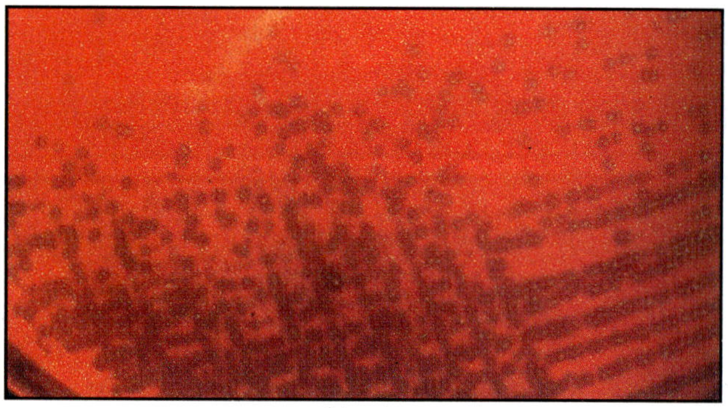

Fig. 30. *Streptococcus pneumoniae* on blood agar showing α-haemolysis.

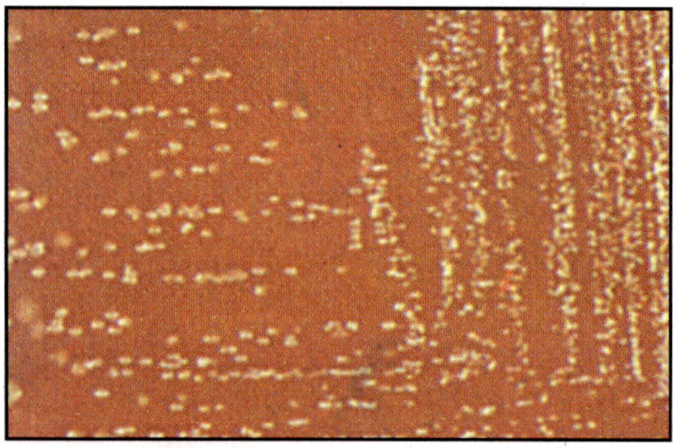

Fig. 31. *Neisseria gonorrhoeae* growing on Thayer-Martin medium.

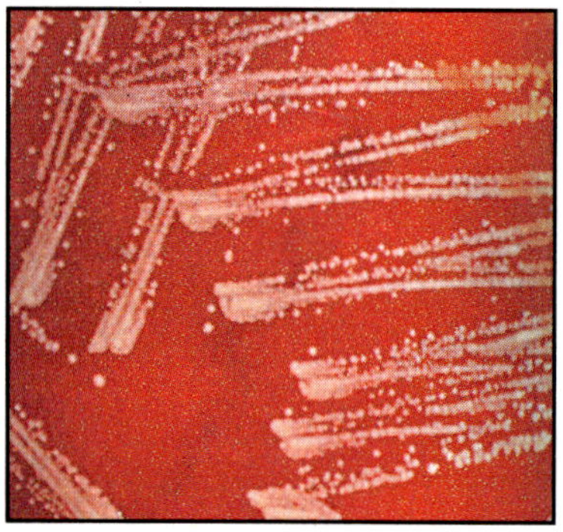

Fig. 32. *Corynebacterium diphtheriae* growing on blood agar.

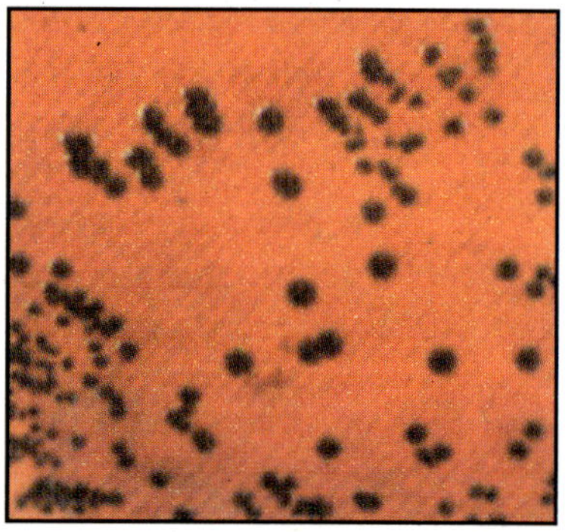

Fig. 33. *C. diphtheriae* showing black colonies on blood tellurite agar.

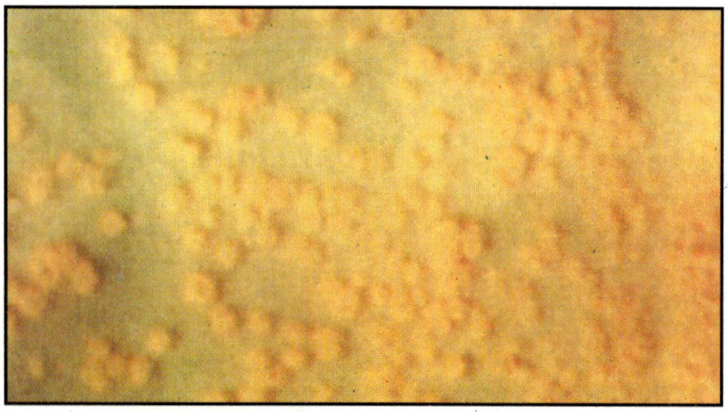

Fig. 34. Growth of *Mycobacterium tuberculosis* on Lowenstein-Jensen medium.

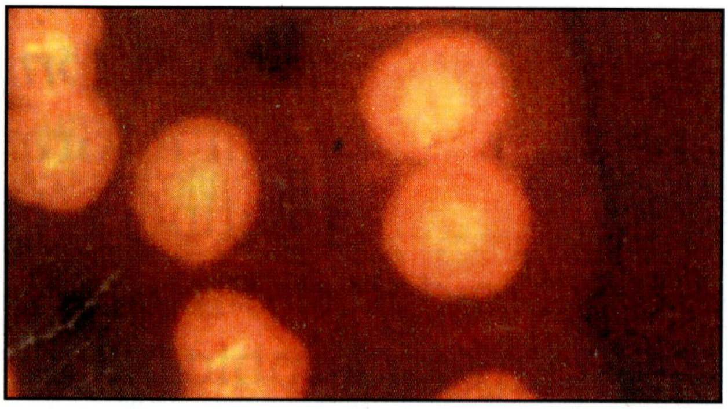

Fig. 35. *Clostridium perfringens* showing double zone haemolysis on blood agar.

PLATE VII

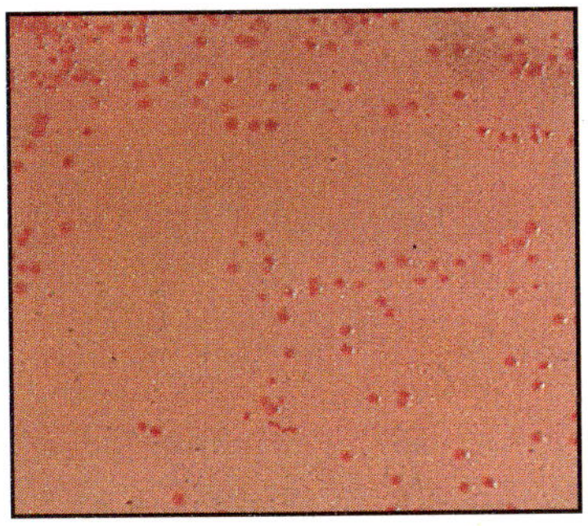

Fig. 36. *Escherichia coli* showing lactose fermenting colonies on MacConkey agar.

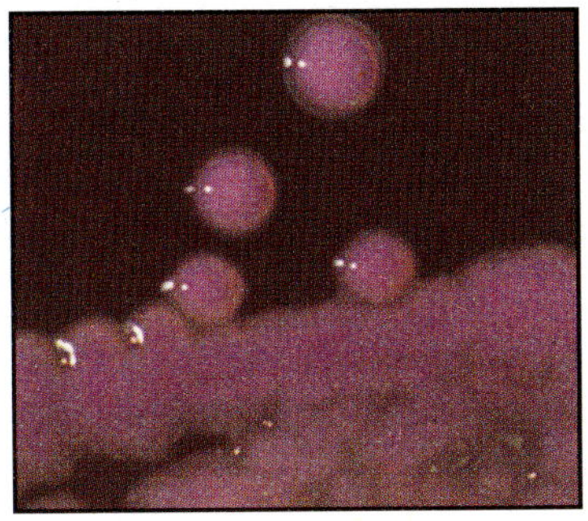

Fig. 37. *Klebsiella* spp. showing mucoid lactose fermenting colonies on MacConkey agar.

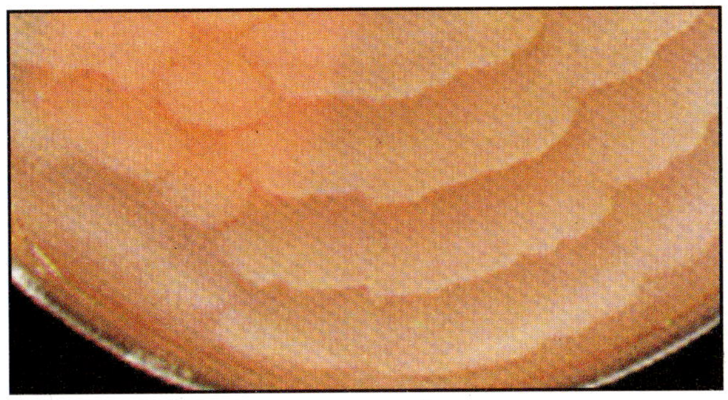

Fig. 38. *Proteus mirabilis* showing swarming on blood agar.

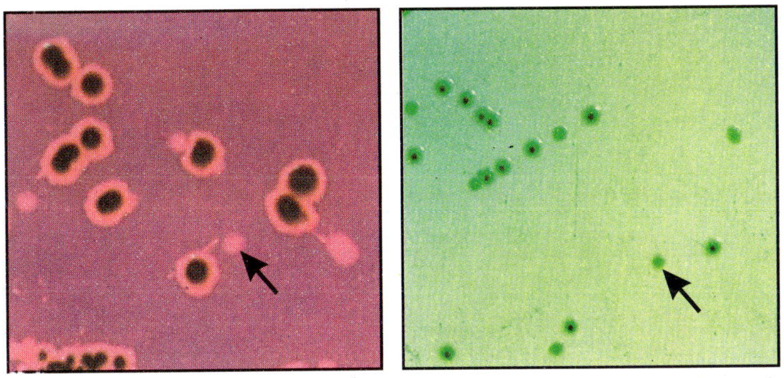

Fig. 39. *Shigella* spp. showing red colonies on xylose lysine deoxycholate agar (left), and green colonies on Hektoen enteric agar(right).

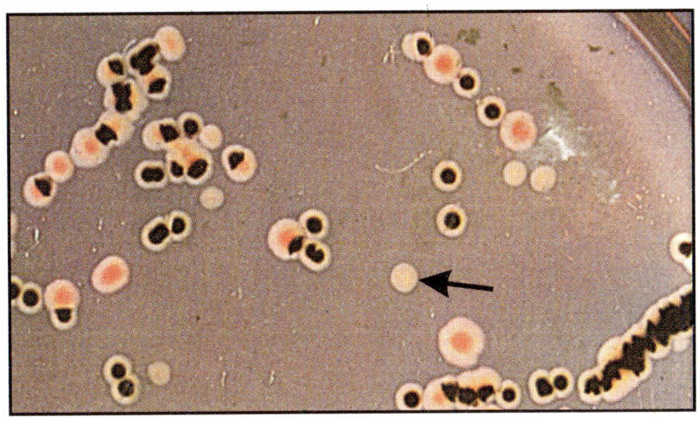

Fig. 40. *Shigella* spp. showing colourless colonies on *Salmonella-Shigella* agar.

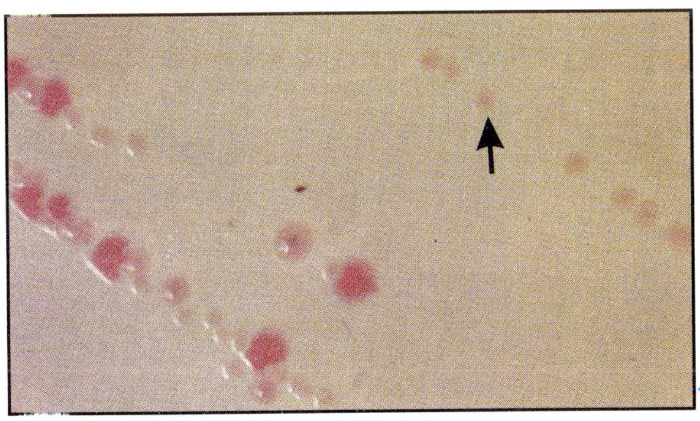

Fig. 41. *Salmonella* Typhi showing colourless colonies on MacConkey agar.

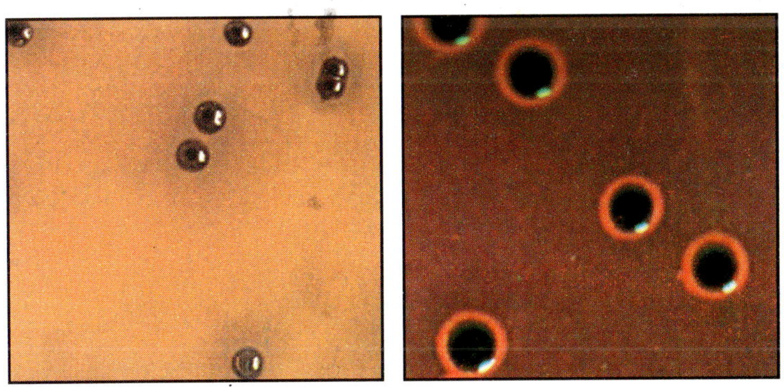

Fig. 42. *Salmonella* Typhi showing black colonies on Wilson and Blair's medium (left), and red colonies with black centres on XLD agar (right).

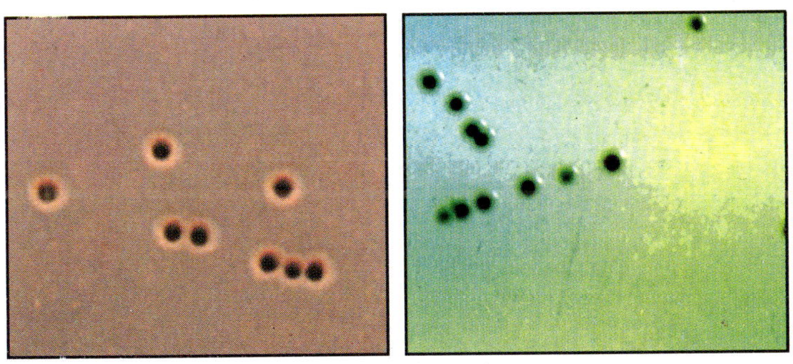

Fig. 43. *Salmonella* spp. showing colourless colonies with black centres on Salmonella-Shigella agar (left), and green colonies with black centres on Hektoen enteric agar (right).

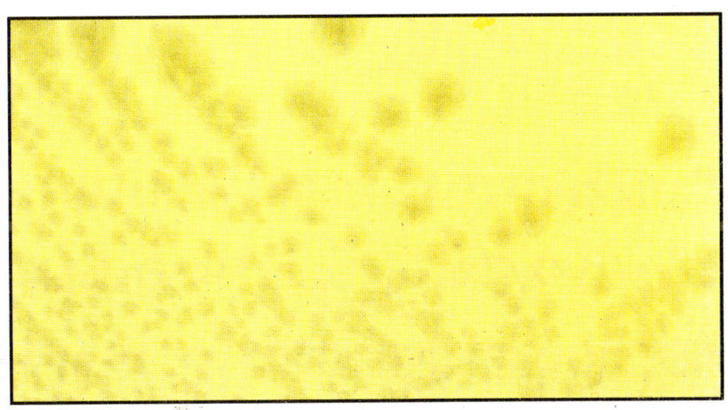

Fig. 44. *Pseudomonas aeruginosa* growing on nutrient agar.

PLATE VIII

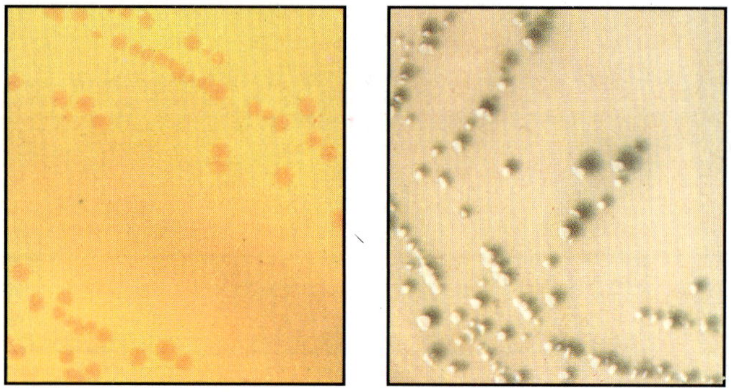

Fig. 45. *Vibrio cholerae* showing yellow colonies (left), and *V. parahaemolyticus* showing green ones (right) on TCBS agar.

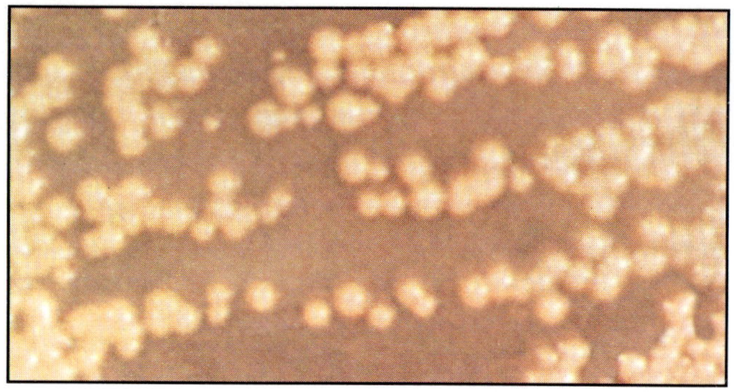

Fig. 46. *Candida albicans* showing colonies on Sabouraud's dextrose agar.

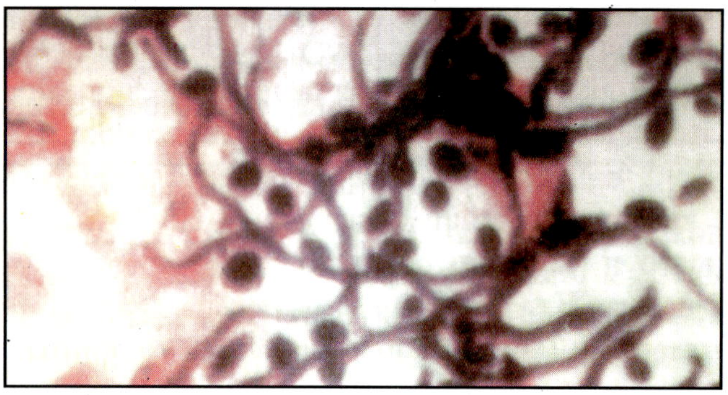

Fig. 47. Gram-stained smear of *Candida* showing budding yeast cells and pseudohyphae.

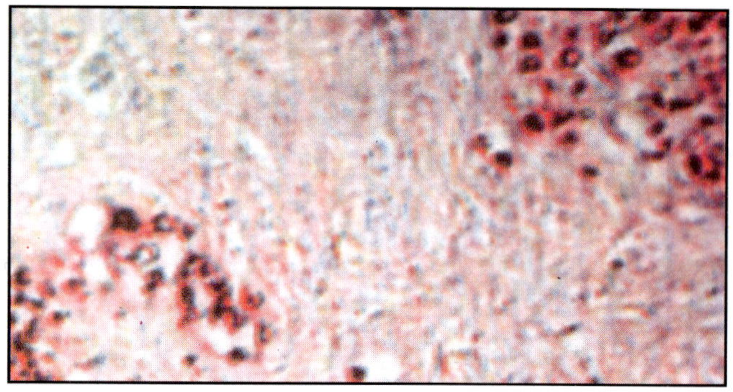

Fig. 48. Cryptococci stained with Mayer's mucicarmine stain. The capsule is stained red in colour.

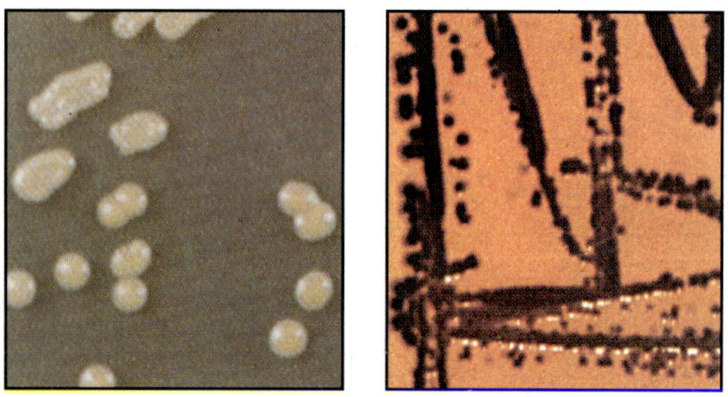

Fig. 49. *Cryptococcus neoformans* growing on SDA (left), and showing black colonies on niger seed agar (right).

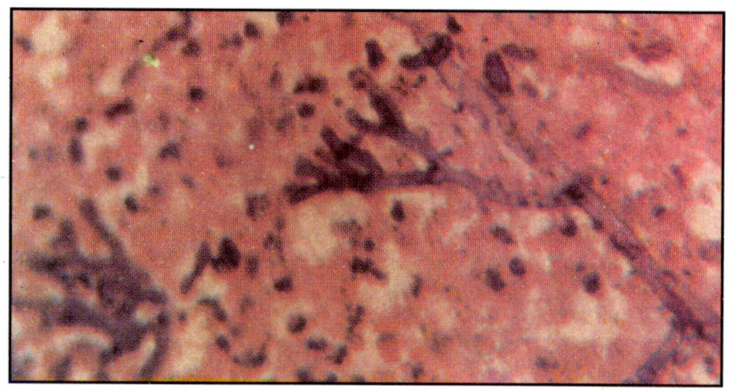

Fig. 50. *Aspergillus* showing septate hyphae with characteristic dichotomous branching.

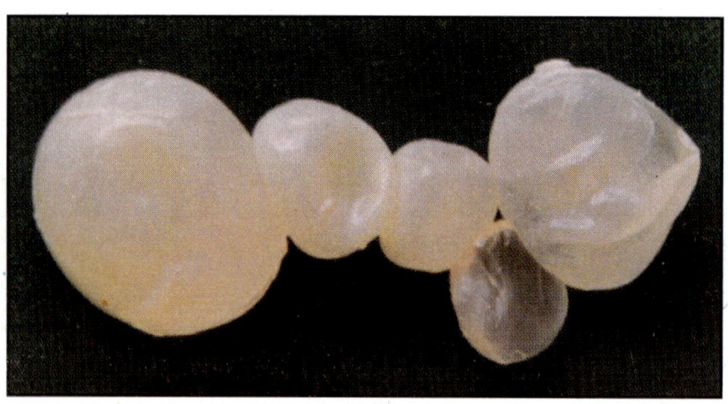

Fig. 51. Hydatid cysts.

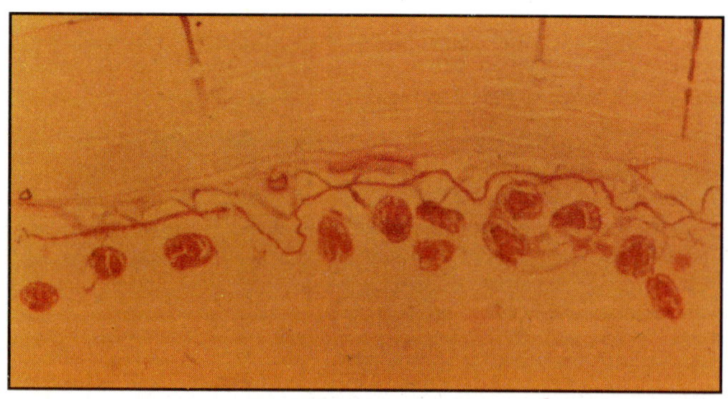

Fig. 52. Hydatid cyst showing laminated hyaline ectocyst, endocyst and scolices.

Contents

Contents

PART–1

General Bacteriology

Contents

Practical 1

The Compound Microscope

Instructions while using microscope

- Keep the microscope on a table that is free from vibration.
- Do not place it in front of a window where bright day light will cause unwanted glare. Use artificial light for the microscope.
- Always adopt a comfortable posture.
- Identify all the essential parts of microscope (Fig. 1.1).
- If wearing spectacles, take care to avoid contact between the eyepiece and the spectacles.
- Before using a microscope, first clean the eyepiece, objectives, condenser lens and stage.

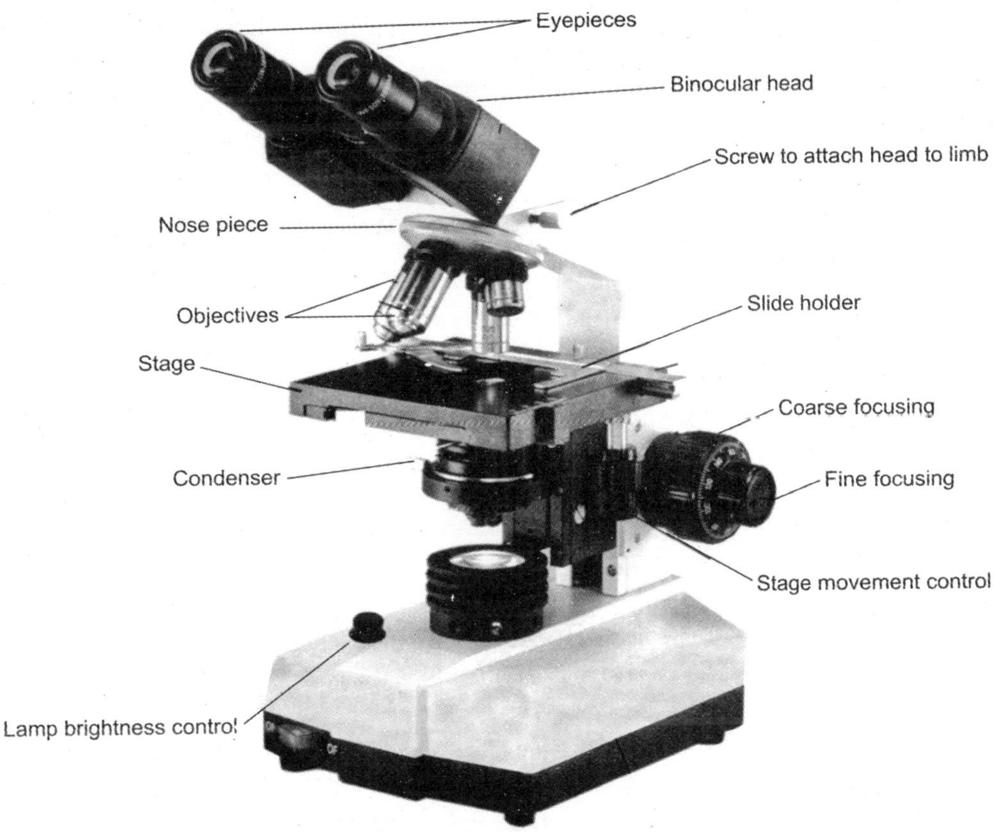

Fig. 1.1. Binocular microscope.

- Make sure the underside of the slide and surface of the stage are completely dry and clean.
- Use plane side of the mirror.
- Raise the condenser to within 1 mm of its top-most position and open the iris.
- Adjust the light by moving up and down the condenser and also by closing or opening the iris diaphragm.
- Obtain the best possible image by adjusting the condenser iris:
  - for the 10X objective, close the iris about two thirds.
  - for the 40X objective, open the iris more.
  - for the 100X objective, open the iris fully and use 7X eyepiece with this objective.
- Always focus the slide first with the 10X objective followed by 40X or 100X as required. While changing the objective from one power to another, always hear the click sound otherwise objective may not be in place for proper illumination.
- Move the objective carefully downwards using the coarse focusing knob until the lens is near the slide. Then looking through the eyepiece, move the objective slowly upwards with the coarse adjustment knob until the image comes into the view. Then adjust with the fine adjustment knob until image is clear.
- Focus continuously to avoid organisms and structures in different planes being missed or misidentified.
- Use a cover-slip when examining the specimen with the 10X or 40X objective.
- Put a drop of oil on the dried slide, when using 100X objective. Always check that the oil has been added to the smear side of the slide. Mark the smear side of the slide with glass marker.
- The oil-immersion objective must be cleaned after use with a tissue paper. Use xylene to remove the dried oil.
- Always move the 100X objective to one side when inserting and removing slide to prevent scratching of the front lens of the objective.
- Keep the microscope under a plastic cover after the work is over. If the microscope is to be moved, do not hold it by the body limb. It should be lifted by the upright limb.

Discussion

1. **Define resolving power of microscope.**
   This is defined as the ability to distinguish clearly two points that are close together within the structure of a particular object.

2. **What is magnification?**
   The degree of enlargement of the object is known as magnification.

3. **What is the limit of resolution of naked eye, light microscope and electron microscope?**
   These are 200 μm, 0.2 μm and 0.3 nm for naked eye, light microscope and electron microscope respectively.

4. **Enumerate various compound microscopes.**
   - Light microscope
   - Phase-contrast microscope
   - Dark-ground (Dark-field) microscope
   - Fluorescence microscope
   - Electron microscope

5. **What are the major advantages of microscopes?**
   - Microscopes are used to visualize very small objects which are not seen clearly with naked eye.
   - They are used for diagnosing many diseases especially those caused by parasites.

6. **Why oil is used while examining the object under oil-immersion lens?**
   Oil has same refractive index as that of glass. Due to the presence of oil, light is not refracted outwards but passes straight into the objective and helps in visualization of the object (organisms).

7. **Which side of mirror is used for reflecting light up through the condenser?**
   Plane mirror

8. **Which agent should be used to clean the oil-immersion objective?**
   Xylene

9. **How do you differentiate, whether dirt seen in the image is from the objective or eyepiece?**
   Rotate one of the eyepieces, if the dirt also rotates it is in the eyepiece.

10. **What do you suspect if blurred image is seen with 40X objective lens?**
    The objective lens may become contaminated from a wet preparation or may have oil.

11. **How glare is minimized while using microscope?**
    - Adjust the iris diaphragm according to the objective in use.

- Avoid using a large source of illumination than is necessary.
- Do not position a microscope in front of sunlight.

12. **What are the uses of dark-field microscopy?**
Dark-field microscopy is useful for detecting spirochaetes such as:
   - *Treponema pallidum* in the lesions
   - Borreliae in blood
   - Leptospires in urine

13. **Which light is used in fluorescence microscope?**
Ultraviolet light

14. **How do the organisms appear in dark-field microscopy?**
Organisms appear as bright objects against a dark background.

Practical 2

Gram Staining

Introduction

The Gram stain was introduced by Hans Christian Gram, a Danish physician in 1884. This is the most frequently used differential stain that divides bacteria into two major groups: (1) Gram-positive and (2) Gram-negative. Gram staining reaction depends on whether or not the organism resists decolourization with acetone or alcohol after staining with pararosaniline dye and further treatment with mordant (Gram's iodine). Bacteria which resist decolourization and remain dark purple after counterstaining are called Gram-positive bacteria while bacteria which get decolourized and take the light pink colour after counterstaining with safranin, neutral red or dilute carbol fuchsin are called Gram-negative bacteria.

Principle

The exact mechanism of Gram reaction is not known. It may, however be attributed to:

- Gram-positive bacteria have more acidic protoplasm, which may account for their retaining the basic primary dye more strongly than Gram-negative bacteria.
- The violet basic dye and the iodine forms a dye-iodine complex inside both Gram-positive and Gram-negative bacteria but during decolourization, cell membranes (outer membrane of cell wall and cytoplasmic membrane) are dissolved. However, dye-iodine complex is retained in Gram-positive cells by the thick peptidoglycan mesh, whereas it is readily washed out through the very thin peptidoglycan layer remaining in Gram-negative cells after both membranes have been dissolved.

Requirements

Slides
Spirit lamp
Nichrome loop
Glass marker
Normal saline
Distilled water
Cedar-wood oil
Gauge piece
Light microscope

Reagents

- Crystal violet (2%) or methyl violet (0.5%) or gentian violet (1%)
- Gram's iodine

  Iodine crystal 1 g
  Potassium iodide 2 g
  Distilled water 100 ml

Dissolve 2 g potassium iodide in 25 ml water, and then add 1 g iodine. When iodine is dissolved, make up to 100 ml with water.

- Acetone or alcohol
- Safranin (0.1%) or dilute carbol fuchsin (1:10)

Procedure

a. Smear Preparation

1. Take a grease-free clean slide and make an oval-shaped mark at the centre by using a glass marker.
2. Transfer a loopful of liquid culture with a sterile nichrome loop and make a smear in the premarked area on the slide (for solid culture take a loopful of

saline on the slide and emulsify the organisms in an area of 1 cm).

3. Allow the smear to air-dry.
4. Fix the dry smear by passing the slide 3–4 times through the flame quickly with smear side facing up. The smear is said to be fixed when it is just tolerable on the dorsum of hand. Over-heating chars the smear.

b. Staining

1. Place the slide on the staining glass rods.
2. Cover the smear with 2% crystal violet and leave for 1 minute.
3. Wash the slide with Gram's iodine.
4. Cover the smear with Gram's iodine and allow it to act for 1 minute.
5. Drain off the iodine.
6. Decolourize with alcohol or acetone. Acetone is the fastest decolourizer. It is applied to smears for only 2–3 seconds. While alcohol acts more slowly than acetone and should be applied and re-applied for about 1 minute until on tilting the slide from side to side and viewing against a white background, colour is no longer seen to flow out of the preparation.
7. Wash under tap water.
8. Counterstain the smear with dilute carbol fuchsin or 1% safranin for 30 seconds.
9. Wash with water and allow the stained smear to dry in air (or dry with blotting paper).
10. Put a drop of cedar-wood oil on the stained smear and observe under oil-immersion lens (100X) of microscope.

Results

Gram-positive bacteria (Colour Plate I, Fig. 1)	Dark purple
Gram-negative bacteria (Colour Plate I, Fig. 2)	Light pink or red
Yeast cells	Dark purple
Tissue cells	Pink
Red blood cells	Pink
White blood cells	Pink
Nuclei of pus cells	Pink to red
Epithelial cells	Pale red

Uses

1. It helps to differentiate bacteria into two groups i.e. Gram-positive and Gram-negative.
2. This differentiation is helpful in determining the use of subsequent culture media and biochemical tests.
3. On the basis of the shape we can differentiate between cocci and bacilli.
4. It helps in identification of organism on the basis of arrangement e.g. Gram-positive cocci in chains (streptococci) and Gram-positive bacilli with Chinese letter arrangement (*Corynebacterium diphtheriae).*
5. Presence of spore (unstained area) and its position can be determined.
6. It helps in starting antibacterial treatment e.g. cell wall acting antibiotics in case of Gram-positive cocci and broad spectrum antibiotics in case of Gram-negative bacilli.
7. It helps to identify host cells. Presence of host cells such as squamous epithelial cells in respiratory specimen indicates contamination with organisms and cells from the mouth.
8. Presence of inflammatory cells (e.g. phagocytes) are key indicator of an infectious process.

Gram-positive organisms that have lost cell wall integrity because of antibiotic treatment, old age, or action of autolytic enzymes may allow crystal violet to wash out with the decolourizing step and may appear Gram-variable, with some cells staining pink and others staining violet. However, for identification purposes these organisms are considered Gram-positive. On the other hand, Gram-negative bacteria rarely, if ever, retain crystal violet if staining procedure has been properly performed.

Not all bacteria can be seen in the Gram stain. Table 2.1 lists the medically important bacteria that cannot be seen in Gram stain and describes the reason why. The alternative microscopic approach to Gram stain is also given.

Table 2.1. Medically important bacteria that cannot be seen in Gram Stain

Microorganisms	*Reason*	*Alternative microscopic approach*
Mycobacteria including *M. tuberculosis*	Too much lipid in cell wall so dye cannot penetrate	Acid-fast stain
Treponema pallidum	Too thin to see	Dark-field microscopy or fluorescent antibody
Mycoplasma pneumoniae	No cell wall; very small	Giemsa
Legionella pneumophila	Poor uptake of red counterstain	Prolong time of counterstain
Chlamydiae including *C. trachomatis*	Intracellular; very small	Giemsa
Rickettsiae	Intracellular; very small	Giemsa or other tissue stains

Discussion

1. **What are mordants?**

   Mordants are substances used in staining treatment which penetrate into a bacterial cell and help to retain the original dye within the cell (by forming a link between organism and stain).

2. **Can Gram-positive organism appear as Gram-negative?**

   Yes, under following situations it can be so:
   - Overdecolourization of the smear
   - Smear prepared from old cultures
   - Use of iodine solution which is too old (yellow instead of brown)
   - Cell wall damage due to excessive heat fixation of the smear, antibiotic therapy or action of autolytic enzymes

3. **Name few Gram-positive bacilli.**
   - *Corynebacterium*
   - *Clostridium*
   - *Bacillus*
   - *Actinomyces*
   - *Nocardia*
   - *Streptomyces*
   - *Listeria*
   - *Erysipelothrix*

4. **Name Gram-negative cocci.**
   - Meningococci
   - Gonococci
   - *Veillonella*

5. **Differentiate between cell walls of Gram-positive and Gram-negative organisms.**

	Gram-positive	*Gram-negative*
Thickness	Thicker	Thinner
Teichoic acid	Present	Absent
Lipids	Absent /scanty	Present
Aromatic and sulphur containing amino acids	Absent	Present
Peptidoglycan	50–90% of the dry weight of the cell wall	5–10% of dry weight of the cell wall

6. **Name organisms which lack cell wall.**
   - *Mycoplasma*
   - *Ureaplasma*
   - *Spiroplasma*
   - *Anaeroplasma*

7. **Mention few coccobacilli.**
   - *Kingella*
   - *Acinetobacter*
   - *Calymmatobacterium granulomatis*

8. **Mention any organism which occurs in octad pattern.**

   Sporosarcina

9. **Name various decolourizing agents.**

   Acetone, absolute alcohol, acetone-alcohol and iodine-acetone

10. **What are the advantages of fixation of a smear?**
    - The smear gets fixed to the slide.
    - Bacteria gets killed and become non-infectious.

Practical 3

Ziehl-Neelsen Staining

Introduction

Ziehl-Neelsen staining method is used for staining of acid-fast bacilli (AFB). Acid-fastness has been attributed to the high content of lipids, fatty acids and higher alcohols found in acid-fast bacteria. Of the lipids, mycolic acid, a high molecular weight hydroxy acid wax containing carboxyl groups, is the most important because it is acid-fast even in free state. Because of these lipids ordinary aniline dye solutions do not penetrate the cell wall. The staining solution used to stain acid-fast bacilli is prepared by using a strong mordant dye like basic fuchsin with phenol. For penetration of the dye into the bacillus heating of the stain is necessary.

Principle

Basic fuchsin in combination with phenol penetrates the cell wall and stains the bacilli bright red. Once stained they resist decolourization with strong acid. The basic dye in combination with mineral acid forms a yellowish-brown compound which easily comes out of the non-acid-fast bacilli after decolourization but not out of the acid-fast bacilli. Counterstaining with methylene blue is done to form a contrast to red coloured acid-fast bacilli.

Reagents

- Ziehl-Neelsen carbol fuchsin

Basic fuchsin (powder)	5 g
Phenol (crystalline)	25 g
Absolute alcohol (ethanol)	50 ml
Distilled water	500 ml

- Sulphuric acid 20%
- Loeffler's methylene blue 0.5%

Requirements

Same as in practical 2.

Procedure

Smear preparation

1. Take a new, unscratched slide and make an oval-shaped mark (2 cm × 3 cm) at the centre by using a glass marker.
2. Make a smear from blood-tinged or yellow purulent portion of the sputum using a stick in the premarked area.
3. Allow the smear to air-dry for 15–30 minutes.
4. Fix the smear by passing the slide over the flame 3–4 times.

Staining

1. Place the slide on the staining glass rods with the smeared side facing upwards.
2. Pour filtered carbol fuchsin over the slide so as to cover the entire slide.
3. Heat the slide underneath until vapours start rising. Do not allow carbol fuchsin to boil or the slide to dry. Continue the process for five minutes.
4. Wash both sides of the slide with tap water.
5. Cover the slide with 20% sulphuric acid. The red colour of the preparation is changed to yellowish-brown. After about a minute in the acid, wash the slide with water, and pour on more acid. Repeat this process several times. The object of the washing is to remove the compound of acid with stain and allow fresh acid to gain access to the preparation. The

decolourization is finished when, after washing, the film is only faintly pink. Decolourization generally requires contact with sulphuric acid for a total of at least 10 minutes.

6. Counterstain with Loeffler's methylene blue for 15–20 seconds.
7. Wash with water.
8. Place the slide in slide tray and allow it to dry.
9. Put a drop of oil on the stained area and observe under oil-immersion (100X) magnification.

Results

Acid-fast bacilli (Colour Plate I, Fig. 3)	Bright red bacilli against blue background
Pus cells	Blue
Squamous epithelial cells	Blue
Elastic fibres	Blue

Uses

1) Ziehl-Neelsen method of staining is useful in detection of acid-fast organisms.
2) Number of bacilli in the smear may be counted and correlated with infectiousness of the person. This is important for epidemiological purpose.
3) This is useful in following a patient's response to treatment.
4) To know the drug resistance. If organisms fail to decrease after therapy in the smear, the possibility of drug resistance must be considered.

Grading of microscopy smears *(Mycobacterium tuberculosis)*

Examination	*Grading*
> 9 AFB per oil-immersion fields	4+
1–9 AFB per oil-immersion fields	3+
1–9 AFB per 10 oil-immersion fields	2+
1–9 AFB per 100 oil-immersion fields	1+
1 or 2 per 300 oil-immersion fields	Doubt or repeat

How to prevent false positive sputum results?

- Ask the patient to rinse the mouth with water before collecting sputum sample.
- There should not be any food particle or fibre in the sputum sample.
- Use only new, unscratched slides.
- Always use filtered carbol fuchsin.
- Do not allow carbol fuchsin to boil during staining.
- Decolourize adequately with sulphuric acid.
- Never touch the oil-immersion applicator to a slide.
- Always clean the oil-immersion lens after screening each smear.

How to prevent false negative sputum results?

- Make sure that sample contains sputum and not just saliva.
- There should be enough sputum (at least 2 ml).
- Select thick, purulent portions to make the smear.
- Fix the smear with correct length of time.
- Prepare smear with adequate material.
- Stain with carbol fuchsin for 5–7 minutes.
- Do not decolourize with sulphuric acid too intensively.
- Examine every smear for at least five minutes observing at least 100 fields before recording as negative.

Discussion

1. **What do you mean by acid-fastness?**
   Acid-fast bacteria do not stain readily with dilute solutions of dyes. But they, do stain when heated with a strong dye solution, and once stained they resist decolourization even by strong mineral acid.
2. **Name various acid-fast organisms.**
   Tubercle bacilli, lepra bacilli, atypical mycobacteria, *Nocardia* spp., *Legionella micadadei, Rhodococcus* spp., bacterial spores, and oocysts of *Cryptosporidium parvum* and *Isospora belli*
3. **Why tubercle bacilli are acid-fast?**
   Due to the presence of mycolic acid in their cell wall.
4. **Why heating of carbol fuchsin is necessary in Ziehl-Neelsen staining?**
   Heating helps in penetration of dye (carbol fuchsin) through waxy coat surrounding the cell wall of mycobacteria.
5. **What are the other methods of acid-fast staining?**
   - Kinyoun acid-fast stain
   - Fluorochrome stain
6. **Why Kinyoun acid-fast stain method is known as cold method?**
   The Kinyoun stain is known as "cold stain" because the high concentration of phenol in the reagent serves to 'dissolve' the lipid material in the cell wall, allowing penetration of the carbol fuchsin dye without the use of heat.
7. **Which method of staining is most useful screening procedure?**
   Fluorescent dye staining

8. **What are the limitations of acid-fast staining?**
   - Smear must always be correlated with culture results.
   - Organisms other than mycobacteria may demonstrate various degrees of acid-fastness.
   - Rapidly growing mycobacteria may stain poorly or acid-fast variable.

9. **What is the number of bacilli which must be present in the sputum for detection by direct microscopy?**
   Fifty thousand to 100,000 bacilli per ml

10. **What is the minimum number of bacilli which must be present in the sputum for detection by direct microscopy while using standard concentration technique?**
    Ten thousand/ml

11. **Can we use counterstain other than methylene blue?**
    Yes, malachite green may be used.

12. **What is the disadvantage of malachite green?**
    This is a strong counterstain and may mask the presence of AFB.

13. **Can we decolourize the smear with acids other than sulphuric acid?**
    Yes, nitric acid or hydrochloric acid.

14. **What is the role of phenol in carbol fuchsin?**
    It acts as mordant. It also makes the cell surface easily penetrable for basic fuchsin by dissolving fats.

15. **What is the concentration of sulphuric acid used for decolourization of various acid-fast organisms?**

Microorganisms	*Per cent concentration of sulphuric acid*
M. tuberculosis	20
Atypical mycobacteria	20
M. leprae	5
Cryptosporidium	1–5
Nocardia spp.	0.5
Bacterial spores	0.25–0.5

16. **How can you differentiate smegma bacilli present in the urine from *M. tuberculosis*?**
    M. tuberculosis is acid- and alcohol-fast while smegma bacilli (commensals) are only acid-fast.

Practical 4

Albert Staining

Introduction

Albert staining method is commonly used for staining and demonstration of *Corynebacterium diphtheriae*, the causative agent of diphtheria. They are thin, Gram-positive bacilli of varying length with an average size of 3 × 0.3 μm. They frequently possess club-shaped swellings at one or both ends, a characteristic feature, which is responsible for the name of the genus. When dividing, the bacilli snap and bend abruptly and appear as angled pairs or parallel rows of 3 to 4 bacilli (palisades) which resemble Chinese letters.

Principle

The granules consist of long-chain inorganic polyphosphates and because of its characteristic reaction they are termed as **metachromatic granules** or **volutin granules** or **Babes-Ernst bodies**. In unstained wet preparation they appear as round refractile bodies within the bacterial cytoplasm. Most cells contain 2 or 3 of these, and they tend to be on poles. Their presence in thin slender bacilli helps to distinguish *C. diphtheriae* from short, thick plumpy, nonpathogenic diphtheroids which lack them. With Albert stain, the granules stain bluish-black and cytoplasm green.

Requirements

Same as in Practical 2.

Reagents

Albert's stain

Toluidine blue	0.15 g
Malachite green	0.20 g
Glacial acetic acid	1 ml
Alcohol (95%)	2 ml
Distilled water	100 ml

Dissolve the dyes in the alcohol and add to the water and glacial acetic acid. Allow to stand for one day and then filter.

Albert's iodine

Iodine	2 g
Potassium iodide	3 g
Distilled water	300 ml

Procedure

1. Make film, dry in air, and fix by heat.
2. Place the slide on the staining glass rods.
3. Cover the smear with Albert's stain and allow to act for 3–5 minutes.
4. Drain the staining solution, but do not wash.
5. Cover the smear with Albert's iodine and allow to act for 1 minute.
6. Wash with water.
7. Dry with blotting paper and observe under 100X magnification of microscope.

Results

Metachromatic granules (Colour Plate I, Fig. 4)	Bluish-black
Bacillary body or protoplasm	Green

Uses

1. Albert staining is useful in the demonstration of metachromatic granules.

2. Presence of metachromatic granules helps to distinguish *C. diphtheriae* from diphtheroids which lack them.
3. Differentiation of three biotypes of *C. diphtheriae* can be done on the basis of granules.

Discussion

1. **What is the chemical nature of metachromatic granules?**
   The granules consist of long-chain inorganic polyphosphates. It appears that they represent storage depots for materials needed to form high-energy phosphate bonds.
2. **What are the other names of metachromatic granules?**
   Babes-Ernst granules, volutin granules and polar bodies
3. **Why are they called Babes-Ernst granules?**
   Because they were first observed by Babes-Ernst.
4. **On which medium granule formation is best seen?**
   Loeffler's serum slope
5. **How can you differentiate *C. diphtheriae* from diphtheroids on the basis of granules?**
   Diphtheroid bacilli do not exhibit metachromatic granules.
6. **In which biotype of *C. diphtheriae* prominent granulation is seen?**
   Mitis
7. **In which biotype of *C. diphtheriae* few or no granules are present?**
   Gravis
8. **How can you differentiate diphtheroids from biotype gravis?**
   Diphtheroids are arranged in V forms or palisades rather than Chinese letter arrangement. They can also be differentiated on the basis of toxigenicity test and fermentation of starch and glycogen, which are shown by biotype gravis.
9. **What is maximum number of these granules in a single bacillus?**
   Six
10. **What are the other stains devised for demonstration of granules?**
    Neisser's and Ponder's stain
11. **Why are they called corynebacteria?**
    They frequently show club-shaped swellings and hence the name corynebacteria (*coryne* meaning club).
12. **What is the other name of *C. diphtheriae*?**
    Klebs-Loeffler bacillus
13. **In which other organism volutin granules are found?**
    Spirillum volutans

Practical 5

Spore Staining

Introduction

Spores are highly resistant resting forms which occur after a period of vegetative growth. Members of several bacterial genera are capable of forming endospores. The two most common are Gram-positive rods: the aerobic genus *Bacillus* and the anaerobic genus *Clostridium.* The other bacteria known to form endospores are the Gram-positive coccus *Sporosarcina* and possibly the rickettsial agent of Q fever, *Coxiella burnetii.*

Principle

Spores are most simply observed as intracellular refractile bodies in unstained cell suspension or as unstained bodies in Gram stain (Colour Plate I, Fig. 5). The spore wall is relatively impermeable, but dyes can be made to penetrate it by heating the preparation. The same impermeability then serves to prevent decolourization of the spore by a period of alcohol treatment sufficient to decolourize vegetative cells. The latter can finally be counterstained. They are commonly stained with malachite green or modified Ziehl-Neelsen staining (0.25% sulphuric acid as decolourizer).

Malachite green stain for spores (Schaeffer and Fulton method)

Requirements

Same as in practical 2–4.

Reagents

Malachite green 5%
Safranin (0.5%) or basic fuchsin (0.05%)

Procedure

1. Prepare a smear on a clean glass slide, dry it in air and fix it by heat.
2. Cover the smear with malachite green stain and heat gently (till steam rises) by placing the gas flame below the slide for about 5 minutes.
3. Wash under running tap water.
4. Cover the smear with safranin for 1–2 minutes.
5. Wash and dry.
6. Observe under oil-immersion lens.

Results (Colour Plate I, Fig. 6)

Spores	Green
Vegetative bacilli	Red
Lipid granules	Unstained

Uses

1. It helps in identification of spore-bearing organisms.
2. Position of spores can be determined (i.e. central, terminal or subterminal).
3. Morphology of spore can be determined (bulging or nonbulging), spherical or oval.

Discussion

1. **What is the concentration of sulphuric acid used for decolourization of bacterial spores?**
   0.25%
2. **What are the uses of bacterial spores?**
   - Bacterial spores are used as biological control to check the efficiency of sterilization methods :

Method of sterilization	*Biological control*
Hot air oven	*Bacillus subtilis* subsp. *niger*
Autoclave	*Bacillus stearothermophilus*
Ionizing radiation	*Bacillus pumilis*
Ethylene oxide	*Bacillus subtilis*

- Spores vaccine (non-capsulated strain of *Bacillus anthracis*) is used in animals to protect them from anthrax.

3. **By which method spores of all medically important species are destroyed?**
   Autoclaving at 121°C for 10–30 minutes
4. **Compare bacterial spores with fungal spores?**

Bacterial spores	*Fungal spores*
• Method of preservation	• Method of reproduction
• Known as endospores	• Known as asexual and sexual spores
• Highly resistant	• Delicate

Practical 6

Capsule Staining

Introduction

Cell wall in many bacteria is enclosed by a protective gelatinous covering layer. If it is easily washed off and does not appear to be associated with the cell in any definite fashion it is referred to as a slime layer, on the other hand if it appears as discrete, thickened gel around each cell, it is known as capsule. Capsule cannot be stained with ordinary stains like Gram staining. They are demonstrated by negative staining methods, either by the wet-film India ink preparation or by dry-film India ink or nigrosin preparation.

Wet India ink film

This is the simplest and most widely applicable method. In this method capsules are not shrunken, as they are not dried or fixed and hence demonstrated clearly.

Requirements and reagents

Bacterial culture
Glass slide
Cover-slip
Inoculating loop
Spirit lamp
India ink

Procedure

1. Place one loopful of India ink on a perfectly clean glass slide.
2. Emulsify a small portion of bacterial culture in the drop of India ink with the help of a sterile loop.
3. Place a clean cover-slip on the drop of India ink without introducing air bubbles.
4. Press down the cover-slip through a sheet of blotting paper so as to get thin film.
5. Observe under oil-immersion objective (100X magnification).

Result

On microscopical examination with the oil-immersion objective the highly refractile outline of the bacterium is seen. Between the refractile surface-membrane and the dark background of ink particles there is a clear space which represents the capsule (Colour Plate I, Fig. 7). Non-capsulated bacteria do not show this clear zone. The ink particles directly abut the refractile wall and in consequence, these bacteria are not easily seen.

Uses

This method is useful in identification of capsulated organisms.

Discussion

1. **Name capsulated organisms.**
   - *Streptococcus pneumoniae*
   - *Neisseria meningitidis*
   - *Klebsiella pneumoniae*
   - *Haemophilus influenzae*
   - *Yersinia pestis*
   - *Bacillus anthracis*
2. **What are the functions of capsule?**
   - Capsule protects the bacteria from antibacterial agents.

- It inhibits phagocytosis thus contributing to the virulence of bacteria.

3. **Which serological method is used to demonstrate capsule?**
   Quellung reaction or capsule swelling
4. **Briefly describe Quellung reaction.**
   Capsular material is antigenic. So when a suspension of a capsulated bacterium is mixed with its specific anticapsular serum and examined under the microscope, the capsule becomes very prominent and appears 'swollen' due to an increase in its refractivity. This is known as Quellung reaction and is employed for the identification of capsular serotypes.

Practical 7

Motility of Bacteria

Method

Hanging drop method

Introduction

Bacteria are motile with the help of flagella. On microscopic examination of wet-films, motile bacteria are seen swimming in different directions across the field. True motility should be differentiated from passive drifting and Brownian movement.

True motility

The organisms move in different directions and change their position in the field.

Passive drifting

Organisms move in the same direction in a convectional current in the fluid.

Brownian movement

This is a rapid oscillation of bacterium within a very limited area due to bombardment by the water molecules.

Requirements

- Glass slide
- Plasticine ring
- Cover-slip
- Nichrome loop
- Spirit lamp
- Light microscope
- Bacterial culture (suspension)

Procedure

1. Place a small ring of plasticine over a clean glass slide. Alternatively, a slide with concavity may be used.
2. Put a drop of bacterial suspension on a cover-slip.
3. Invert the glass slide over the cover-slip, allowing cover-slip to adhere to the slide.
4. Now turn around the slide so that cover-slip is on the top and drop of bacterial suspension hangs in the centre of plasticine ring from the under surface of cover-slip (Fig. 7.1).
5. Examine under the microscope with condenser lying low. Focus the margin of hanging drop with low power and then swing the objectives to the high power lens (40X magnification) (Fig. 7.2).
6. Observe for motility of bacteria.

Results

- Motile organisms – Detected by the presence of directional motion.
- Non-motile organisms – No movement.

Uses

1. Detection of motility of organisms.
2. Shape, approximate size and general structure can be observed.

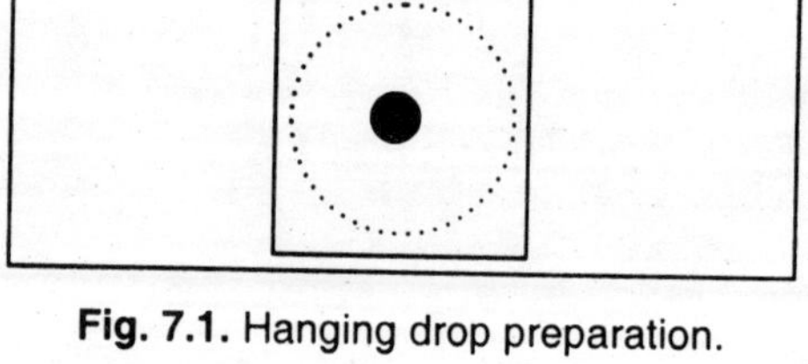

Fig. 7.1. Hanging drop preparation.

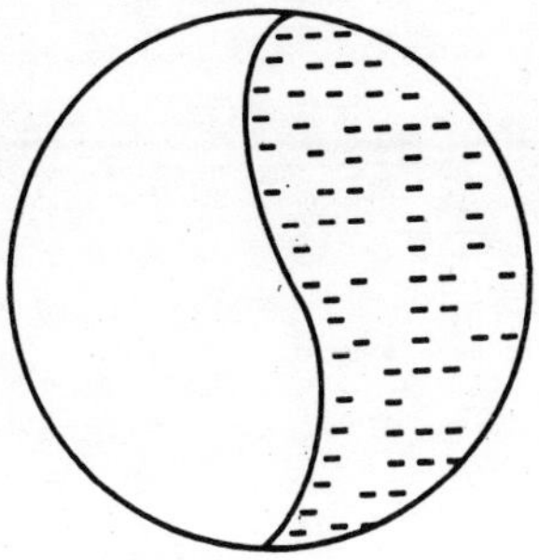

Fig. 7.2. Hanging drop examination under 40X magnification.

3. Type of motility can be observed e.g. darting motility is shown by *Vibrio cholerae*.

Discussion

1. **Enumerate various types of motility giving example.**

Type of motility	*Example*
Darting motility	*Vibrio cholerae*
Very actively motile	*Proteus* spp.
Actively motile	*Escherichia coli*
Tumbling motility	*Listeria monocytogenes*
Gliding motility	*Mycoplasma pneumoniae*
Corkscrew motility	*Campylobacter* spp. & spirochaetes

2. **Name the organs of motility.**
   Flagella

3. **What is the organ of locomotion in spirochaetes?**
   The motility in spirochaetes is due to one or more pairs of axial filaments which run between outer membrane and peptidoglycan layer and are anchored by knobs at both poles.

4. **Name non-motile Gram-positive bacilli.**
   - *Clostridium perfringens*
   - *Bacillus anthracis*

5. **Name other methods of determining motility of bacteria.**
   - Cragie's tube technique
   - Mannitol motility medium
   - Swarming on solid medium

Practical

8

Sterilization

Introduction

Sterilization is defined as the process by which an article, a surface or a medium is freed of all microorganisms including viruses, bacteria, their spores and fungi, both pathogenic and nonpathogenic. The process of sterilization is used in microbiology for prevention of contamination of culture media from bacteria in air, dust, etc. Heat is the most reliable, certain and rapid method of sterilization. There are two types of heat: dry heat and moist heat (Tables 8.1 and 8.2). Dry heat is believed to kill microorganisms by causing destructive oxidation of essential cell constituents. The moist heat causes denaturation and coagulation of proteins.

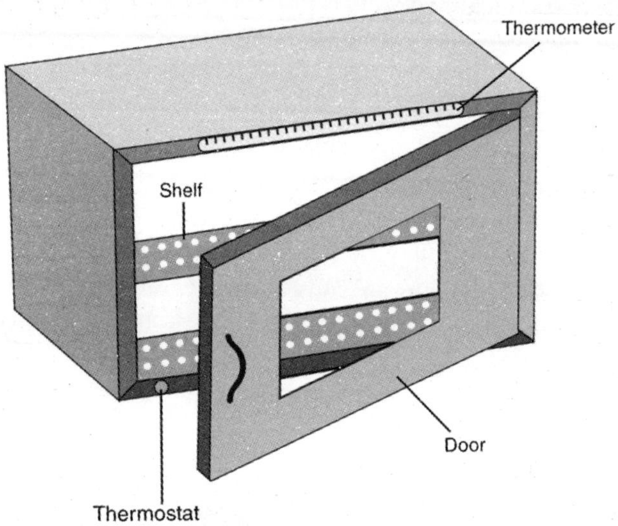

Fig. 8.1. Hot air oven.

Hot air oven

It is a method of choice for sterilization of glassware such as assembled all glass syringes, test tubes, petri dishes, pipettes and flasks, metal instruments such as forceps, scissors and scalpel, materials such as oils, jellies and powders which are impervious to steam and swab sticks packed in test tubes. It is not suitable for materials like fabrics which may be damaged by heat. Hot air oven is electrically heated and is fitted with a thermostat that maintains the chamber air at a chosen temperature and a fan that distributes hot air in the chamber (Fig. 8.1). It must not be overloaded and spaces must be left for circulation of air through the load. Holding time for steriliza-

Table 8.1. Sterilization by dry heat

Mode of sterilization	*Instrument*	*Temperature and time*	*Sterilization of*
Red heat	Bunsen burner	Till red hot	Inoculating wire loops, forceps and spatulas
Flaming	Bunsen burner	Waving through the flame	Scalpel blades, glass slides, mouth of culture tubes and bottles
Hot air	Hot air oven	160°C for 1 hour or 180°C for 20 minutes	Glassware, metal instruments, sealed materials such as oils, greases, dry powder, swab sticks packed in test tubes, etc.

Table 8.2. Sterilization by moist heat

Mode of sterilization	*Instrument*	*Temperature and time*	*Sterilization of*
Below 100°C	Water-bath	56°C for 1 hour or 65–75°C for 10 minutes	Serum, body fluids, vaccines and spatulas
At 100°C	Boiling water-bath	100°C for 10–20 minutes	Glass, metal and rubber items
Steaming at 100°C	Arnold steamer	100°C for 20 minutes on 3 successive days	Culture media containing sugar and gelatin
Above 100°C	Autoclave	121°C for 15–20 minutes	Culture media and aqueous solutions, dressing material, linen, gloves, etc.

tion in hot air oven is one hour at 160°C or 20 minutes at 180°C. It is timed as begining when the thermometer first shows 160°C or 180°C respectively.

Sterilization controls

Two types of controls are available.

Chemical control

A Browne's tube containing red solution is placed within the load. A change of colour of the solution to green indicates proper sterilization.

Biological control

An envelope containing a filter paper strip impregnated with 10^6 spores of *Bacillus subtilis* subsp. *niger* is placed within the load. After sterilization is over, the strip is removed and inoculated into tryptone soy broth and incubated aerobically at 37 °C for five days. No growth of *B. subtilis* subsp. *niger* indicates proper sterilization.

Autoclave

Sterilization by steam under pressure (autoclaving) is suitable for culture media and aqueous solutions, dressing material, linen, gloves, etc. Satisfactory sterilization can be achieved at 15 pounds per square inch (psi) pressure equivalent to 121°C in 15–20 minutes. The laboratory autoclave (Fig. 8.2) consists of a vertical or horizontal cylinder of gun metal or stainless steel in a supporting frame.

The lid is fastened by screw clamps and rendered air tight by asbestos gasket. Lid bears a pressure gauge, and a steam release valve or safety valve. The latter opens and closes when the steam pressure rises or falls the desired level respectively. On its upper part of the side, the autoclave has a discharge tap for air and steam, and an air and steam knob. Heating is done by electricity. Water is added on the bottom of the autoclave. Above this is a perforated shelf on which articles to be sterilized are placed. The lid is closed, discharge tap is opened and safety valve is adjusted to the required pressure. As heating continues, the steam and air mixture escapes. When all the air from inside the autoclave has been removed then the discharge tap is closed. Steam pressure rises inside and when it reaches the desired set level (15 psi) the safety valve opens and excess steam escapes. From this point the holding time (15 minutes) is counted. When the holding time is over, the heating is stopped and autoclave allowed to cool till pressure gauze indicates that inside pressure has reached to the atmospheric pressure. The discharge tap is now opened and air allowed to enter the autoclave. The lid is now opened and the sterilized articles removed.

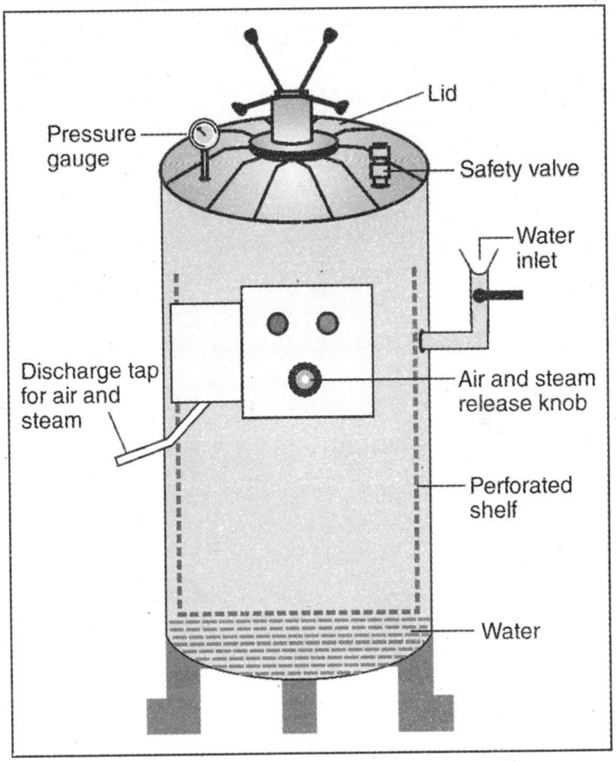

Fig. 8.2. Autoclave.

Biological control

Bacillus stearothermophilus. It is processed as in case of hot air oven. However, incubation is done at 56°C.

Chemical control

A Browne's tube containing red solution as in case of hot air oven.

Discussion

1. **Define the term sterilization.**

   Sterilization is defined as the process by which an article, a surface or a medium is freed of all microorganisms including viruses, bacteria, their spores and fungi, both pathogenic and nonpathogenic.

2. **Define the term disinfection.**

   Disinfection is a process of destruction or removal of organisms capable of giving rise to infection. Disinfectants are capable of killing vegetative bacteria, fungi, viruses and rarely bacterial spores.

3. **What do you mean by antiseptic?**

   A disinfectant that is applied to living tissue is referred to as an antiseptic.

4. **What is the mechanism of sterilization by dry heat?**

   Dry heat is believed to kill microorganisms by causing destructive oxidation of essential cell constituents.

5. **What is the mechanism of sterilization by moist heat?**

   The moist heat causes denaturation and coagulation of proteins. When steam condenses on cooler surface, it releases its latent heat and raises the temperature of its surface. If spores are present, steam condenses on them and increases their water content leading to hydrolysis and breakdown of bacterial proteins.

6. **What is the holding time for sterilization in hot air oven?**

   Holding time for sterilization in hot air oven is one hour at 160°C or 20 minutes at 180°C.

7. **Name biological control to check the efficacy of hot air oven.**

   Bacillus subtilis subsp. *niger* (NCTC 10075 or ATCC 9372)

8. **What do you mean by low temperature steam-formaldehyde (LTSF) sterilization?**

   Items which cannot withstand heat at 100°C may be disinfected by steam at sub-atmospheric pressure at a temperature of 75°C with formaldehyde vapour. This is known as LTSF sterilization.

9. **How many methods of pasteurization are there?**

   Holder method : The temperature employed is 63°C for 30 minutes.

   Flash method : 72°C for 20 seconds followed by rapid cooling to 13°C

10. **Which organism may survive pasteurization by holder method?**

    Coxiella burnetii, causative agent of Q fever

11. **What do you mean by tyndallization or intermittent sterilization?**

    One single exposure to steam for 90 minutes ensures complete sterilization but for culture media containing sugar and gelatin, which may get decomposed on long heating, an exposure of 100°C for 20 minutes on three consecutive days is employed. This is known as tyndallization.

12. **Why an exposure of three consecutive days is required in tyndallization?**

    First exposure to steam kills vegetative bacteria and any spore present, being in a favourable medium, will germinate and will be killed on the subsequent occasion.

13. **Enumerate items which can be sterilized in hot air oven.**

    - Glassware
    - Metal instruments
    - Liquid paraffin
    - Jellies
    - Powders
    - Swab sticks packed in test tubes

14. **Why steam above 100°C or saturated steam is more efficient sterilizing agent than hot air?**

    - It provides greater lethal action of moist heat.
    - It is quicker in heating up the exposed articles.
    - It can penetrate easily porous materials such as cotton-wool stoppers, paper and cloth wrappers, bundles of surgical linen, and hollow apparatus.

15. **Enumerate articles which are sterilized in autoclave.**

    - Culture media
    - Aqueous solutions
    - Dressing material
    - Linen
    - Gloves

16. **What temperature and pressure are required for sterilization by autoclaving?**

    Sterilization can be achieved at 15 pounds per square inch (psi) pressure equivalent to 121°C in 15–20 minutes.

17. **Name one biological control to check the efficacy of autoclave.**

    Bacillus stearothermophilus (NCTC 10003 or ATCC 7953)

18. **Enumerate physical agents of sterilization.**
    - Sunlight
    - Drying
    - Heat
    - Filtration
    - Radiation
19. **Which method of sterilization can kill all bacterial spores?**
    Autoclaving at 121°C for 10–30 minutes
20. **Name one steam sterilizer.**
    Koch or Arnold steam sterilizer
21. **Enumerate media which are sterilized in an inspissator.**
    Lowenstein-Jensen's medium and Loeffler's serum slope
22. **What temperature and time are required for sterilization in an inspissator?**
    80–85°C for half an hour on three successive days.
23. **Why hot air oven is allowed to cool after sterilization process?**
    It is allowed to cool for about two hours before the door is opened, since the glassware may crack due to sudden or uneven cooling.
24. **How do you sterilize inoculating loop or wire?**
    They are sterilized by holding them vertical in a bunsen burner flame until red hot.
25. **What is the method of sterilization of serum or body fluids?**
    Serum or body fluids containing coagulable proteins can be sterilized by heating for one hour at 56°C in a water-bath.
26. **Define cold sterilization.**
    Sterilization of disposable items by ionizing radiations or ethylene oxide is known as cold sterilization.

Practical 9

Liquid Culture Media

Introduction

Culture media are essential for isolation and identification of microorganisms which help in diagnosis and treatment of infectious diseases.

Classification of media

Culture media have been classified as under:

1. Solid, semi-solid and liquid media.
2. Simple (basal), complex, synthetic, defined, semi-defined, and special media. Special media are further divided into enriched, selective, enrichment, indicator or differential, sugar media and transport media.
3. Aerobic media and anaerobic media.

Commonly used liquid culture media

1. Peptone water
2. Nutrient broth
3. Sugar media
4. Bile broth and glucose broth
5. Cooked meat broth (CMB)
6. Hiss's serum water
7. Buffered glycerol saline
8. Selenite F broth
9. Venkatraman-Ramakrishnan medium (VR medium)
10. Tetrathionate broth

1. Peptone water

This is a sugar free basal medium. It contains peptone (10 g), sodium chloride (5 g) and distilled water (1000 ml). It is a watery colourless solution with pH 7.4–7.6 (Colour Plate II, Fig. 8A).

Uses

- It is a liquid basal medium used for preparation of sugar media.
- It is mainly used for culturing a large number of non fastidious organisms.
- Peptone water is used for testing indole production.
- It is also used for studying the motility of organisms.
- It is used for cultivation and as an enrichment medium for *Vibrio cholerae* by raising the pH to 8.4 (alkaline peptone water).

2. Nutrient broth

This is a basal medium for the preparation of other media. It contains meat extract, infusion or digest (10 g), peptone (10 g), sodium chloride (5 g) and distilled water (1000 ml). It is a clear, straw coloured transparent fluid with pH 7.4–7.6 (Colour Plate II, Fig. 8B). Three types of nutrient broths can be prepared:

- *Meat infusion broth*
- *Meat extract broth*
- *Meat digest broth*

Uses

- It is more nutritious than peptone water and may be used for growth of fastidious organisms.
- This medium is routinely used for culture of common bacteria.
- It is used as a basal medium for preparation of cooked meat broth employed for cultivation of anaerobes.
- It is used for preparation of bile broth and glucose broth.
- It is used for testing of disinfectants.

3. Sugar media

A large variety of carbohydrates are used for identification of organisms. The basal medium for sugars is peptone water. It contains 1% sugar (glucose, lactose, mannitol, sucrose) in a sterilized peptone water (pH 7.2–7.4). It also contains 1% Andrade's indicator. Various other indicators having a pH range between 6–8 such as bromothymol blue and neutral red can also be used. Sugar media are dispensed in tubes containing inverted Durham's tube (Colour Plate II, Fig. 8C). Various sugar media in tubes can be identified by incorporating cotton-wool stoppers of different colours.

Uses

- Sugar media are used for testing the sugar fermentation reaction for identification of various organisms (fermentation is indicated by development of red colour due to the production of acid).
- Gas producing bacteria can be identified by observing air in Durham's tube.

4. Bile broth and glucose broth

These are primary culture media for blood culture. These contain nutrient broth (100 ml), glucose/bile (1 g) and sodium citrate (0.2 g) (Colour Plate II, Fig. 8D & E). In most of the patients with septicaemia and pyrexia of unknown origin, the organisms present in the blood are very few, so large amount of blood (5–10 ml) is required. Blood itself contains antibacterial substances. Hence for diluting these antibacterial substances 10-fold dilution of the blood in the medium (50–100 ml) is required. The addition of liquoid (sodium polyanethol sulphonate) counteracts the bactericidal action of blood.

Uses

- Bile broth is used for isolation of *Salmonella* spp. from blood of the patients suffering from enteric fever.
- Glucose broth is used for isolation of pyogenic organisms from blood e.g. streptococci from cases of bacterial endocarditis.

5. Cooked meat broth

This medium is used for the isolation of anaerobic organisms. It contains meat cooked in sodium hydroxide and then filtered and squeezed. The meat particles in the medium act as a reducing agent and provide anaerobic atmosphere. The meat particles are dispensed in sterile test tube to give a tall column (approximately 2.5 cm). Sterile nutrient broth is added to give a column of 5 cm above the meat particles. A tall column of meat is essential because the conditions are anaerobic only when the column of meat is sufficiently high. Addition of paraffin on the top of nutrient broth further seals off the atmospheric oxygen (Colour Plate II, Fig. 8F).

Uses

It is used :

- For isolation of anaerobic organisms.
- As a transport medium for anaerobic organisms.
- To distinguish proteolytic clostridia from saccharolytic. In CMB, saccharolytic clostridia produce acid and gas but they do not digest the meat. The culture may have a slightly sour smell and the meat is often reddened. On the other hand, proteolytic clostridia produce blackening of meat, decompose it and reduce it in volume with the formation of foul-smelling products.
- For preservation of stock cultures of aerobic organisms e.g. streptococci.

6. Hiss's serum water

It consists of 1 part of ox serum and 3 parts of peptone water.

Uses

It is used for biochemical reactions of organisms requiring serum for growth e.g. neisseriae, corynebacteria, etc.

7. Buffered glycerol saline

This medium is purple-pink in colour (Colour Plate II, Fig. 8G) and dispensed in 6 ml amount in universal container.

8. Selenite F broth

It contains sodium hydrogen selenite (4 g), peptone (5 g), lactose (4 g), disodium hydrogen phosphate (9.5 g) , sodium dihydrogen phosphate (0.5 g) and distilled water (100 ml) (Colour Plate II, Fig. 8I). This medium is sterilized by steaming at 100°C for 20 minutes.

Uses

- This is an enrichment medium for the isolation of *Salmonella* and *Shigella*.

9. Venkatraman-Ramakrishnan medium (VR medium)

This medium contains crude sea salt (20 g), peptone (5 g) and distilled water (100 ml). It is dispensed in screw-capped bottles in 10–15 ml amounts. About 1–3 ml stool is to be added to each bottle.

Uses

- This is used as transport or holding medium for *Vibrio cholerae*. In this medium vibrios do not multiply but remain viable for several weeks.

10. Tetrathionate broth

It contains thiosulphate solution, iodine solution, phenol red, calcium carbonate and nutrient broth. This medium should be used within 24 hours of preparation.

Uses

- This medium is used as an enrichment medium for *Salmonella* and *Shigella*.
- **Brilliant green tetrathionate broth:** This broth can be prepared by addition of 0.001% brilliant green to this medium (Colour Plate II, Fig. 8H).

Discussion

1. **What are the advantages of liquid media?**

   In liquid media rapid growth of organisms is obtained. These are used for:
   - Biochemical tests
   - Antibiotic sensitivity tests
   - Studying motility of bacteria
   - For bulk cultures for the preparation of antigens and vaccines

2. **What are the disadvantages of liquid media?**
   - The growth of organisms does not exhibit characteristic appearances. However, pigment production, as in case of *Pseudomonas aeruginosa*, can be easily detected.
   - Individual organism cannot be identified from a mixture containing different organisms.

3. **What is the reducing agent in cooked meat broth?**

   Meat particles act as reducing agent.

4. **Name various reducing agents used in culture media.**

   Glucose (0.5–1%), ascorbic acid (0.1%), cysteine (0.1%) and sodium thioglycollate (0.1%)

5. **Define enrichment medium.**

   When a substance is added to a liquid medium which inhibits the growth of unwanted bacteria and favours the growth of wanted bacteria it is known as enrichment medium.

6. **Mention few enrichment media.**

   Tetrathionate broth and selenite broth for *Salmonella* and *Shigella*, and alkaline peptone water for *Vibrio cholerae*.

Practical 10

Solid Culture Media

Introduction

Robert Koch described means of cultivating bacteria on solid media. Most solid media are solidified by adding agar (a long-chain polysaccharide gelling agent obtained from certain seaweeds). A concentration of 1–2% usually yields a suitable gel. The melting and solidifying points of agar are not the same. At the concentration normally used, most bacteriological agars melt at about 95°C and solidify only when cooled to about 42°C. It does not melt at 37°C (incubation temperature of most pathogenic bacteria) – a property that makes it a suitable solidifying agent for culture media. Most of the culture media are sterilized by autoclaving at 121°C for 15 minutes. Nutrients that are damaged by autoclaving are sterilized separately by filtration, etc. The sterilized agar base is then melted in the steamer and cooled to about 45–50°C followed by addition of heat-labile ingredients but once these are added the medium must at once be poured into petri dishes because it cannot be remelted without damaging the heat-sensitive ingredients. Solid media are used to obtain isolated colonies of organisms.

Commonly used solid media

1. Nutrient agar
2. Blood agar
3. Chocolate agar
4. MacConkey agar
5. Loeffler's serum slope
6. Lowenstein-Jensen medium
7. Sabouraud's dextrose agar
8. Mueller-Hinton agar

1. Nutrient agar

It is a solid basal medium for routine use. It is pale yellowish (Colour Plate II, Fig. 9A) dispensed in petri dishes and test tubes.

Uses

- It is used for growth of common pathogenic organisms.
- It acts as basal medium for the preparation of other media e.g. blood agar, milk agar, salt agar, etc.
- It is used for antibiotic sensitivity testing.
- It is used for demonstration of pigment production in staphylococci and *Pseudomonas*.
- Semi-solid nutrient agar (0.2–0.5% agar) is used for demonstrating motility (Craigie's tube method).
- Concentrated nutrient agar (4–6%) is used for inhibiting the swarming of *Proteus* species.

2. Blood agar

It contains 7–10% sheep blood in nutrient agar. It is red coloured opaque medium contained in petri dishes (Colour Plate II, Fig. 9B). It is a widely used enriched medium in bacteriology.

Uses

- It is used for demonstrating haemolytic property(α, β and γ) of organisms.
- It is useful for growth of most of the pathogens.
- It is used for testing the drug sensitivity of *Haemophilus influenzae* and *Neisseria* species.
- It is used for preparation of chocolate agar.

3. Chocolate agar(heated blood agar)

This medium is more enriched medium than blood agar. It is prepared by heating 10% of sterile blood in sterile nutrient agar. Melt the agar, cool it in a water-bath at 75°C, add the blood and allow the medium to remain at 75°C, mixing the blood and agar by gentle agitation from time to time until the blood becomes chocolate-brown in colour, within about 10 minutes. Then pour in petri dishes. Alternatively it can also be prepared by simply heating the blood agar plates at 55°C by placing in an incubator for 1–2 hours. It is identified by its typical chocolate colour (Colour Plate II, Fig. 9C).

Uses

- This medium is used for the culture of *Neisseria,* pneumococci, *Haemophilus influenzae*, etc.

4. MacConkey agar

MacConkey agar is a differential or indicator medium used for the culture of Enterobacteriaceae group of organisms. It is transparent, pink red in colour and is dispensed in petri dishes (Colour Plate II, Fig. 9D). Presence of bile salt in the medium inhibits the growth of non intestinal organisms. Lactose with an indicator neutral red distinguishes the lactose fermenting coliforms from non-lactose fermenting organisms. Fermentation of lactose by organisms results in acid production which is indicated as pink colour colonies when the indicator is neutral red.

Uses

- It is a useful medium for the culture of the organisms of family Enterobacteriaceae.
- It differentiates lactose fermenting organisms from non-lactose fermenting organisms.
- It can be used as a selective medium for *Salmonella* spp. by the addition of brilliant green.

5. Loeffler's serum slope (LSS)

It contains 3 parts of ox, sheep or horse serum and 1 part sterile glucose broth (1%). It is white opaque medium with small amount of water of condensation. It is dispensed in McCartney bottle as a slope (Colour Plate II, Fig. 9E).

Uses

- This is used for cultivating *Corynebacterium diphtheriae*.
- Growth of *C. diphtheriae* on this medium is rapid (6–8 hours).
- Metachromatic granules of *C. diphtheriae* are well formed in this medium.
- The water of condensation is used for testing the toxigenicity in guinea-pig.

6. Lowenstein-Jensen medium

It contains eggs, malachite green, mineral salt solution (asparagine, glycerol, magnesium sulphate, magnesium citrate, distilled water and potassium dihydrogen phosphate). It is green opaque slope dispensed in McCartney bottle (Colour Plate II, Fig. 9F). 0.75% glycerol enhances the growth of human tubercle bacillus, but glycerol at this concentration is inhibitory to *Mycobacterium bovis* so it fails to grow on this medium. However, when the concentration of the glycerol is reduced to 0.5%, it still improves the growth of *M.tuberculosis* but generally does not inhibit the growth of *M. bovis*. Malachite green inhibits the growth of organisms other than mycobacteria and provides a colour contrast while eggs serve both as enrichment and solidifying agent.

Uses

- It is used for cultivation and isolation of mycobacteria including *Mycobacterium tuberculosis* and atypical mycobacteria.
- It is used for differentiation between human and bovine types of tubercle bacilli.
- It is used for drug sensitivity testing of tubercle bacilli.

7. Sabouraud's dextrose agar

This is a selective medium for the cultivation of fungi. It is pale, semitransparent slope dispensed in large test tubes with pH 5.4 (Colour Plate II, Fig. 9G). Its low pH, high sugar content and incorporation of penicillin and streptomycin prevents the growth of bacteria, and cycloheximide inhibits the growth of contaminating fungi.

Uses

- It is used for cultivation of fungi.
- Sensitivity to antimycotic drugs may be determined in this medium.

8. Mueller-Hinton agar

It contains beef infusion (300 ml), casein hydrolysate (17.5 g), starch (1.5 g), agar (20–30 g) and distilled water (1000 ml). Presence of starch in the medium acts as a colloidal agent against the toxic substances produced during the growth.

Uses

- This medium is used for antibiotic sensitivity testing of most pathogens.
- It is also used for the isolation of pathogenic *Neisseria* species.

Discussion

1. **What are the advantages of solid media?**
   - Bacteria produce discrete visible growth (colonies) with distinct colonial morphology.
   - Different organisms form well-separated colonies from a mixed culture.
   - They exhibit many other characteristic features such as pigment production or haemolysis.

2. **What do you understand by the term enriched media?**

   In these media substances like blood, serum and egg are added to basal medium to increase the nutritious value e.g. blood agar, chocolate agar, Loeffler's serum slope, etc.

3. **Define indicator medium or differential medium.**

   When a substance is added into a medium which would produce a visible change in the medium following the growth of a particular organism, it is designated as indicator or differential medium e.g. MacConkey's medium.

4. **Define selective medium.**

   When a substance is added to a solid medium which inhibits the growth of unwanted bacteria but permits the growth of wanted bacteria it is known as selective medium e.g. Lowenstein-Jensen medium for the isolation of *Mycobacterium tuberculosis.*

5. **What are the advantages of agar?**
   - Agar does not add to the nutritive properties of the medium and is not affected by the growth of bacteria.
   - The melting (95°C) and solidifying (42°C) points of agar are not the same, therefore, heat-labile ingredients can be added to sterilized agar base at 45–50°C.
   - Agar does not alter the pH of the medium.
   - Agar can be added to any nutrient liquid medium if the advantages of a solid medium are desired.

6. **What is the advantage of low pH and high sugar content in Sabouraud's dextrose agar?**

   It prevents bacterial contamination.

7. **What do you mean by term "hard agar"?**

   To prepare a solid medium usually 1–2% agar is used, if the concentration is raised to 6% it is called hard agar.

8. **What is the concentration of agar in semi-solid agar?**

   0.2–0.5%

9. **Which blood is preferred for preparing blood agar plates?**

   Sheep blood is preferred because the haemolysis is better visualized and moreover it does not have any toxic substances which can suppress the growth of bacteria.

10. **Name any medium containing serum.**

    Loeffler's serum slope

11. **Name few media containing egg.**
    - Dorset egg medium
    - Lowenstein-Jensen medium
    - NIH medium

12. **How much medium should be poured in a 100 mm petri dish?**

    Medium should be poured to a depth of 4 mm (25 ml).

Practical 11

Collection and Transportation of Specimen

Collection and transportation of specimens

Blood

- Should be drawn under aseptic conditions.
- Disinfect the skin over the vein with tincture iodine and spirit and wait for a minute.
- Draw out 5 ml of blood for one blood culture bottle containing 50 ml of medium. For pediatric age group, 1 ml blood in 10 ml of medium in McCartney bottle (Fig. 11.1A) may be added.
- Collect blood during early stages of disease since the number of bacteria is higher in acute and early stages of disease.
- Collect blood during paroxysm of fever since the number of bacteria is higher at high temperature in patients with fever.
- In the absence of antibiotic administration, 99% culture positivity can be seen with three blood cultures.
- Transport the specimen to the laboratory. If not possible keep in incubator or at room temperature. Do not refrigerate.

Urine

- Mid-stream urine sample is collected after giving proper instructions to the patient.
  a) Clean the genitalia properly (in case of male, retract the prepuce, clean it with sterile normal saline. In case of female, wash perineum and periurethral area with soap and water).
  b) Collect a "clean-catch" mid-stream urine sample in a sterile bottle (Fig. 11.1B).

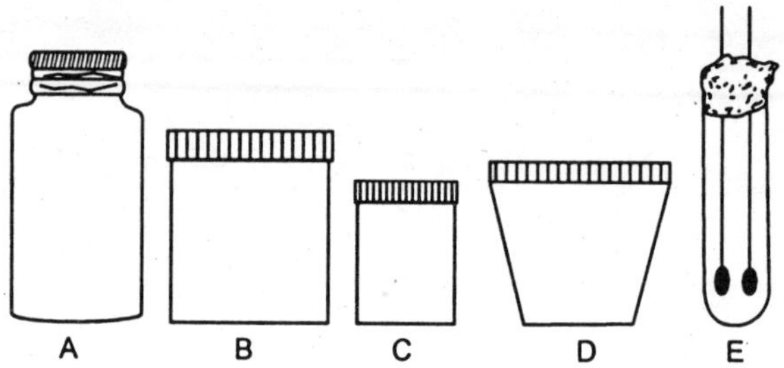

Fig. 11.1. (A) McCartney bottle, (B) Urine/stool container, (C) CSF container, (D) Sputum container, (E) Throat swabs.

- Transport immediately to the laboratory. If a delay of more than 1–2 hours is unavoidable, refrigerate at 4°C.
- In catheterized patients, do not collect urine from collection bag or after opening the closed drainage. Clean the area over the collecting tubes and puncture with the help of a sterile needle and syringe and draw out the sample.
- Suprapubic aspiration under aseptic condition may be done in infants.

Cerebrospinal fluid (CSF)

- Collect CSF in a screw-capped sterile container (Fig. 11.1C) under aseptic conditions.
- Immediately transport to the laboratory and process.
- If delay in processing is inevitable then store it at 37°C.
- Do not refrigerate.

Sputum

- Collect the sputum in a wide-mouthed container, which is preferably disposable, made up of clear thin plastic, unbreakable and leak-proof container (Fig. 11.1D).

- Ask the patient to rinse the mouth with plain water and then inhale deeply 2–3 times, cough up deeply and spit in the sputum container by bringing it close to the mouth. If the patient has difficulty in coughing sputum, postural drainage and appropriate physiotherapy often cause exudate to move in the bronchi and stimulate productive coughing.
- Make sure the sputum sample is of good quality and not just the saliva. A good sputum sample is thick, purulent and sufficient in amount (2–3 ml).
- Sputum sample may be refrigerated up to 3–4 hours.

Throat swab

- Two swabs should be collected (Fig. 11.1E).
- Depress the tongue with a tongue blade.
- Swab the inflammed area of the throat, pharynx or tonsils with a sterile swab taking care to collect the pus or piece of membrane.
- Transport in a sterile transport tube.

Pus and other discharge

- Do not apply antiseptic before collection.
- Clean with normal saline.
- In case of discharge, 1–2 ml of sample is collected in a sterile penicillin vial.
- If swabs are collected, 2 swabs in a sterile container should be collected (one for direct microscopic examination and the other for culture).

Bone marrow

- Decontaminate the skin overlying the site from where specimen is to be collected with tincture iodine and spirit.
- Aspirate 1 ml or more of bone marrow by sterile percutaneous aspiration.
- Collect in a sterile screw-capped tube.
- Immediately transport to the laboratory.

Stool

- Should be collected in early stage of disease and prior to treatment with antimicrobials.
- Do not collect the specimen from bed pan.
- Should not be contaminated with urine.
- Collect 1–2 g sample in a wide-mouthed clean container (Fig. 11.1B).
- If mucus or flakes are present, these must be included.
- If possible, submit more than one specimen on different days.
- The fresh stool specimen must be processed within 1–2 hours of passage.
- If delay is unavoidable then store it at 2–8°C.

Rectal swab

- Collect the swab only if stool collection is not possible.
- Insert swab at least 2.5 cm beyond the anal sphincter so that it enters the rectum.
- Rotate it once before withdrawing.
- Transport in Cary-Blair or other transport medium.

Catheters and tips

- Mark the junction of skin and catheter.
- Withdraw the catheter a little and cut it at about 1 cm distal to the mark.
- Send 5 cm length of the catheter in a sterile container.
- Transcutaneous part is a better sample than the tip in case of long catheters.

Discussion

1. **Name few transport media.**
   - Cary-Blair medium
   - Amies medium
   - Stuart's medium
2. **What is the advantage of transport media?**
   They preserve the viability of bacteria (pathogen) during transport without allowing their multiplication.
3. **Which is the most suitable sample for the diagnosis of urinary tuberculosis?**
   Fifty to 100 ml early morning urine (EMU) is the most suitable specimen.
4. **Why CSF sample should not be refrigerated?**
   Refrigeration of CSF sample tends to kill *Haemophilus influenzae*.
5. **What is the best condition for storage of CSF?**
   The specimen is best kept in an incubator at 37°C.
6. **Why do you collect two swabs?**
   One swab is for making film and the other for seeding culture.

7. **In which clinical situations blood culture is requested?**

Blood culture is requested mainly in two clinical situations:

- Septicaemia or bacteraemia suggested by presence of fever, shock or other signs and sýmptoms occurring in association with a known or suspected local infection such as sepsis in surgical wound, puerperal sepsis, pneumonia, meningitis, osteomyelitis or endocarditis.
- Pyrexia of unknown origin (PUO)

8. **Describe the characteristic features of pus due to different organisms.**

Causative organisms	*Characteristic features of pus*
Staphylococcus aureus	Thick creamy
Streptococcus pyogenes	Watery and straw coloured
Proteus spp.	Fishy smell
Pseudomonas spp.	Sweet, musty odour and often a blue pigmentation
Anaerobes	Offensive putrid smell
Actinomycetes	Sulphur granules
Fungi	Black or brown granules

Practical

12

Cultivation of Bacteria

Introduction

For the cultivation of bacteria, clinical specimens are inoculated on to various culture media. Inoculation is carried out with platinum or nichrome loops of different gauges. Nichrome has oxidizing properties and hence in some of the tests where this property of bacterium is to be tested (e.g. oxidase test), platinum loop, instead of nichrome should be used. The loop is sterilized by holding it vertically in the flame of burner so that the whole length of wire becomes red hot. It is allowed to cool down before it touches any material suspected to be having bacteria to avoid the heat killing of the organisms.

Culture Methods

- Streak culture
- Lawn culture
- Stroke culture
- Stab culture

Requirements

- Inoculating loop/wire
- Marker
- Peptone
- Nutrient agar medium
- Incubator
- Blood culture bottle
- Spirit lamp
- Light microscope
- Pipettes

Streak culture

This method is routinely employed for the isolation of bacteria in pure culture from clinical specimen. Owing to the high cost of platinum, loops for routine use are made of nichrome, No. 24 SWG with internal diameter 2–4 mm. One loopful of the specimen is smeared thoroughly over area A (Fig. 12.1), on the surface of a well dried plate, to give a well inoculum or 'well'. The loop is re-sterilized and drawn from the well in 2 or 3 parallel lines on the fresh surface of the medium (B). This process is repeated as shown (C, D, E), care being taken to sterilize the loop, and cool it on unseeded medium, between each sequence. On incubation, growth may be confluent at the site 'well', but becomes progressively thinner, and well separated colonies are obtained over the final series of streaks.

Lawn culture

Lawn cultures are prepared by flooding the surface of the plate with a liquid culture or suspension of bacteria and pipetting off the excess inoculum or by applying a swab

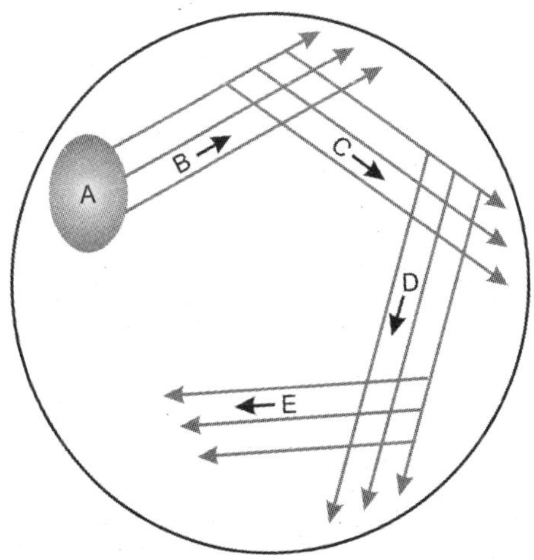

Fig. 12.1. Streak culture.

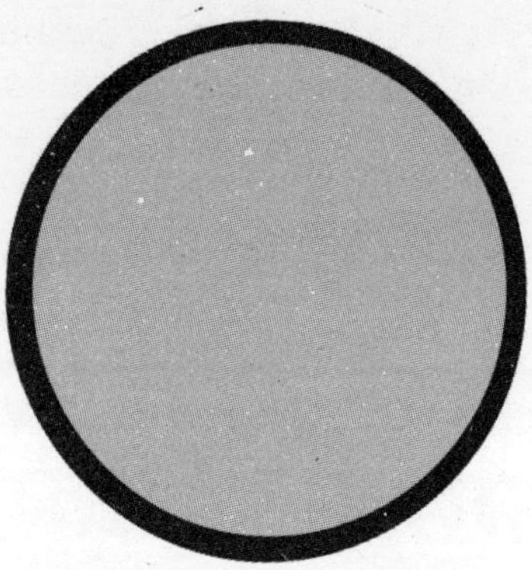

Fig. 12.2. Lawn culture.

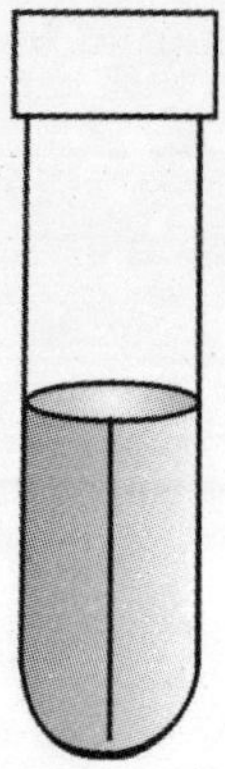

Fig. 12.4. Stab culture.

soaked in the bacterial culture or suspension (Fig. 12.2). After incubation, lawn culture provides a uniform surface growth. It is useful for antibiotic susceptibility testing by disc diffusion method and bacteriophage typing.

Stroke culture

Stroke culture is made in tubes containing agar slope or slant. Slopes are seeded by lightly smearing the surface of agar with loop in zig-zag pattern taking care not to cut the agar (Fig. 12.3). It is used for obtaining pure growth for slide agglutination and other diagnostic tests.

Stab culture

Stab cultures in solid media (nutrient, gelatin or glucose agar) are inoculated by plunging the charged wire into the centre of the medium and withdrawing it in the same line to avoid splitting the medium (Fig. 12.4). These are employed mainly for demonstration of gelatin liquefaction and for the maintenance of stock cultures.

Uses

The purpose of cultivation is to grow the organism and isolate it in pure form which helps in further identification of the organism, antibiotic sensitivity testing, phage typing and serotyping, etc.

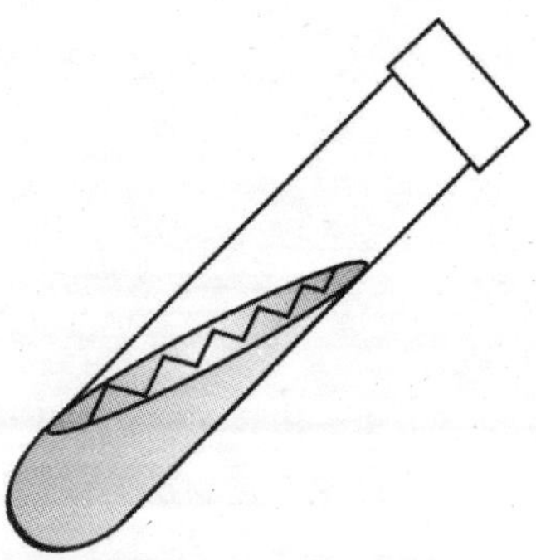

Fig. 12.3. Stroke culture.

Discussion

1. **For which test platinum loop must be used and why?**
   When oxidizing property of a bacterium is to be tested e.g. oxidase test, platinum loop must be used, as nichrome has oxidizing property.
2. **Which method is preferred for obtaining isolated colonies?**
   Streak culture
3. **Describe the order in which solid media should be inoculated.**
   Inoculate media without inhibitors, followed by indicator and then selective media.
4. **Which culture method is used for the maintenance of stock cultures?**
   Stab culture
5. **Name organisms in which incubation is done in an atmosphere with added carbon dioxide (CO_2).**
   Brucella abortus, pneumococci, gonococci, capnophilic streptococci. They are known as capnophilic organisms.
6. **What is the concentration of CO_2 required for the incubation of capnophilic organisms?**
   Five to ten per cent
7. **How do you provide this 5–10% CO_2?**
   - Candle jar
   - CO_2 jars
   - CO_2 incubators (capnoeic incubators)
   - CO_2 generating kits

8. **What precaution should be observed for incubating liquid media in CO_2 environment?**
   Screw caps on containers of liquid media must not be tight and should preferably be replaced by a closure that allows entry of CO_2.

9. **What are the characters to be studied while examining the growth on solid media?**
   Size, shape, surface, elevation, edges, opacity, consistency, emulsifiability in water or saline, pigment production and haemolysis.

10. **Which culture method is used for antibiotic sensitivity testing by disc diffusion method?**
    Lawn culture

Practical 13

Identification of Organisms (Biochemical Reactions)

Introduction

Most important duty of a medical microbiologist is isolation and accurate identification of disease causing orga-nism from the morbid material and its antibiotic susceptibility. Clinical material is inoculated on to a solid medium in such a way so as to ensure isolated discrete colonies. Enriched, enrichment, selective and differential media, depending upon the organism suspected, are emplo-yed. Selective growth conditions i.e. presence or absence of oxygen and presence of CO_2, etc. are also employed keeping in view the organisms suspected. The culture plates are incubated at optimum temperature.

Identification of the isolate is carried out by following tests

- Examination of stained and unstained smears of the morbid material.
- Isolation in pure culture on appropriate culture me-dia.
- Study of macroscopic (colonial characters) and mi-croscopic morphology of the isolate.
- Biochemical reactions.
- Serotyping, biotyping, bacteriocin typing, phage typ-ing, etc.
- Animal pathogenicity.
- Nucleic acid probes and polymerase chain reaction (PCR).
- Antimicrobial susceptibility testing.

Requirements

- Bacterial cultures
- Inoculating loop/wire
- Peptone water
- Glucose phosphate broth
- Kovac's reagent
- Methyl red reagent
- Potassium hydroxide and α-naphthol in absolute al-cohol
- Simmon's medium or Koser's medium
- Nitrate broth
- Sulphanilic acid
- α-naphthylamine
- Christensen's medium
- Lead acetate filter paper strip
- 10% H_2O_2
- 1% oxidase reagent (tetramethyl-p-phenylene-di-amine dihydrochloride)
- Zinc powder
- Phenylalanine agar
- 10% ferric chloride
- Potassium cyanide
- Sugar media
- Spirit lamp
- Incubator

Biochemical reactions

A large number of biochemical tests can be employed for the identification of different bacteria. These include :

1. Indole test

Certain bacteria possessing enzyme tryptophanase, degrade amino acid trytophan to indole, pyruvic acid and ammonia.

Method

- Inoculate peptone water with the test organism and incubate at 37°C for 48–96 hours.
- Add 0.5 ml of Kovac's reagent and shake gently.
- A red colour in the alcohol layer indicates a positive reaction. Indole is extracted upward by amyl or isoamyl alcohol and forms red coloured ring by forming a red coloured complex with paradimethylaminobenzaldehyde. Negative test will show yellow coloured ring (colour of Kovac's reagent) (Colour Plate III, Fig. 10A).

2. Methyl red (MR test)

This test detects the production of sufficient acid by fermentation of glucose so that pH of the medium falls and it is maintained below 4.5.

Method

- Inoculate the test organism in glucose phosphate broth (5 ml) and incubate at 37°C for 2–5 days.
- Add 5 drops of 0.04% methyl red.
- Mix and read the result immediately. If test is negative after 2 days repeat it after 5 days.
  Positive test : Bright red colour (Colour Plate III, Fig. 10B).
  Negative test : Yellow colour.

3. Voges-Proskauer test

Many bacteria ferment carbohydrates with the production of acetyl methyl carbinol (acetoin). In the presence of potassium hydroxide (KOH) and atmospheric oxygen, acetoin is converted to diacetyl, and α-naphthol serves as a catalyst to form a red complex (Colour Plate III, Fig. 10C).

Method

- Inoculate test organism in glucose phosphate broth and incubate at 37°C for 48 hours.
- Add 1 ml KOH and 3 ml of 5% solution of α-naphthol in absolute alcohol.
- Shake the tube for aeration.
  Positive test : Pink colour (2–5 minutes) which becomes crimson in 30 minutes.
  Negative test : Yellow colour.

4. Citrate utilization

This test is used to study the ability of an organism to utilize citrate as a sole source of carbon for the growth. Liquid (Koser's) and solid (Simmon's) media containing citrate as a sole source of carbon can be used. Solid medium contains bromothymol blue as indicator. Citrate utilization results in alkaline pH that turns the indicator from green to blue (Colour Plate III, Fig. 10D).

Method

- Inoculate the test organism with the help of straight wire into either of these media.
- Incubate at 37°C for 24 hours.
  Positive test : Liquid medium : Turbidity
  Solid medium : Appearance of growth and blue colour.
  Negative test : Liquid medium : No turbidity
  Solid medium : No growth and original green colour.

5. Nitrate reduction test

This test detects the production of enzyme nitrate reductase which reduces nitrate to nitrite or free nitrogen gas. Nitrite combines with the test reagent to form diazo red dye (Colour Plate III, Fig. 10E).

Method

- Inoculate test organism in 5 ml of nitrate broth.
- Incubate at 37°C for 96 hours.
- Add 0.1 ml test reagent (equal volume of 0.8% sulphanilic acid and 0.5% α-naphthylamine in 5N acetic acid mixed just before use).
  Positive test : Red colour.
  Negative test : Yellow colour.

6. Urease test

This test detects the ability of an organism to produce urease enzyme. This enzyme converts urea into ammonia and CO_2. Ammonia makes the medium alkaline and phenol red indicator changes to purple pink colour (Colour Plate III, Fig. 10F).

Method

- Inoculate test organism on the entire slope of Christensen's medium (contains urea, phenol red and agar).
- Incubate at 37°C and examine after 4 hours, and after overnight incubation.
  Positive test : Purple pink colour.
  Negative test : Original colour of the medium.

7. Hydrogen sulphide production

This test detects the ability of a few organisms to produce hydrogen sulphide from sulphur containing amino acids.

Method

- Suspend lead acetate filter paper strip between cotton plug and the tube.
- Incubate at 37°C for 24 hours.

  Positive test : Blackening of filter paper strip (Colour Plate III, Fig. 10G).

  Negative test : Original colour of paper strip.

8. Catalase test

This test detects the presence of enzyme catalase which catalyzes the release of oxygen from hydrogen peroxide (H_2O_2).

Method

- Take a drop of 10% H_2O_2 on clean glass slide.
- Pick up a colony to be tested from nutrient agar plate with the help of a glass rod.
- Dip the glass rod in the drop of H_2O_2.

  Positive test : Production of gas bubbles (Colour Plate III, Fig. 10H).

  Negative test : No gas bubbles.

9. Oxidase test

This test depends on the presence , in bacteria, of certain oxidases that catalyze the oxidation of reduced tetra-methyl-p-phenylene-diamine dihydrochloride (oxidase reagent) by molecular O_2.

Method

- Put a drop of freshly prepared 1% solution of reagent on a piece of filter paper.
- Now rub a few colonies of test organism on it with the help of a glass rod.

  Positive test: Purple colour (Colour Plate III, Fig. 10I).

  Negative test : No purple colour.

  Alternatively, pour oxidase reagent over the colonies of test organism on the culture plate. The colonies of oxidase-positive organism rapidly develop a deep purple colour.

10. Motility test

This test detects motile organisms.

Method

- Inoculate test organism in a test medium (agar concentration 0.4% or less to allow free spread of organisms) by a single stab.
- Incubate at 37°C for 24 hours.

  Positive test : Movement away from stab line or a hazy appearance throughout the medium indicates motile organism (Colour Plate III, Fig. 10J).

  Negative test: Bacterial growth accentuated along stab line; surrounding medium remains clear.

11. Potassium cyanide test

This test detects the ability of an organism to grow in the presence of potassium cyanide.

Method

- Inoculate test organism in peptone buffered water containing 1 in 13,000 concentration of potassium cyanide.
- Incubate at 37°C for 24–48 hours.

  Positive test : Development of turbidity in the medium indicates the ability of the organism to grow in presence of potassium cyanide (Colour Plate III, Fig. 10K).

  Negative test : No turbidity.

12. Sugar fermentation test

This test detects the ability of an organism to ferment various sugars. This test also detects the production of gas.

Method

- Inoculate test organism in different sugar media (glucose, lactose, mannitol, sucrose, etc.) containing Andrade's indicator.
- Incubate at 37°C for 24 hours.

  Positive test : Red or pink colour (production of acid changes the colour of the medium). Gas, if produced collects in Durham's tube (a small tube which is kept inverted in the tube containing sugar medium) (Colour Plate III, Fig. 10L).

  Negative test : Original yellow colour.

13. Phenylalanine deaminase test

This test detects the ability of an organism to produce enzyme phenylalanine deaminase that deaminates phenylalanine to phenylpyruvic acid.

Method

- Inoculate test organism in agar slant of medium containing DL-phenylalanine.
- Incubate at 37°C for 18–24 hours.
- Add 4–5 drops of 10% solution of ferric chloride reagent.
  Positive test : Green colour (phenylpyruvic acid reacts with ferric chloride to give green colour) (Colour Plate III, Fig. 10M).
  Negative test : No green colour.

Discussion

1. **Enumerate oxidase-positive organisms.**
   - *Neisseria*
   - *Pseudomonas*
   - *Aeromonas*
   - *Vibrio*
   - *Alcaligenes*
   - *Campylobacter*
2. **What precautions should be taken for doing oxidase test?**
   - Solution of oxidase reagent must be fresh.
   - Platinum loop or glass rod should be used, as traces of iron catalyze the reaction and give false positive result.
   - Growth should not be picked up from medium containing catalase e.g. blood agar.
   - Colour development should be seen within 5–10 seconds.
3. **What precautions should be taken for doing citrate test?**
   - Citrate medium should not be inoculated with liquid medium containing growth. On the other hand a part of a colony is picked up with a straight wire and inoculated.
   - Keep the inoculum light, since dead organisms can serve as source of carbon, producing a false positive reaction.
4. **Which indicators are used in Simmon's citrate medium and Christensen's medium?**
   Bromothymol blue in Simmon's citrate medium and phenol red in Christensen's medium
5. **Why red coloured ring is formed at the top in the indole positive test?**
   Indole formed in the medium is extracted upward by amyl or isoamyl alcohol and reacts with paradimethylaminobenzaldehyde to form red coloured ring.
6. **Enumerate organisms showing positive phenylalanine deaminase test.**
   - *Proteus* spp.
   - *Morganella* spp.
   - *Providencia* spp.

Practical 14

Antimicrobial Susceptibility Testing

Introduction

Antimicrobial susceptibility tests are very essential step for the proper treatment of infectious diseases. These are performed on bacteria isolated from clinical specimens. These are not performed on bacteria that are isolated from the anatomic sites of which they are normal inhabitants and on those that are predictably sensitive to the antimicrobial agents commonly used to treat infections caused by these bacteria. Group A β-haemolytic *Streptococcus,* for example, is not routinely tested because it is universally sensitive to penicillin, the drug of choice in treating infections caused by this bacterium. These tests are of two types:

1. Diffusion methods

- Kirby-Bauer disc diffusion method
- Stokes disc diffusion method

2. Dilution methods

- Broth dilution method
- Agar dilution method

Requirements

- Mueller-Hinton agar/broth
- Antibiotic discs
- Bacterial culture
- Straight wire/loop
- Turbidity standard (0.5 McFarland)
- Incubator
- Control strains (ATCC/NCTC)
- Swab sticks

Kirby-Bauer disc diffusion method

- Sterile Mueller-Hinton agar is poured into plates.
- When the agar has solidified, dry the plates for 10–30 minutes at 37°C by placing them in an upright position in the incubator with the lids tilted.
- To prepare the inoculum from the primary culture plate, touch the tops of 5–10 similar appearing colonies with a straight wire or loop.
- Inoculate them in a suitable broth medium. Incubate at 35–37°C for 4–6 hours when the growth is considered to be in logarithmic phase.
- The density of the organisms is adjusted to approximately 10^8 colony forming units (cfu)/ml by comparing its turbidity with that of 0.5 McFarland opacity standard (0.5 standard contains 9.95 ml of 1% sulphuric acid and 0.05 ml of 1% barium chloride). Proper adjustment of the turbidity of the inoculum is essential to ensure that the resulting lawn of growth is confluent or almost confluent.
- Within 15 minutes after adjusting the turbidity of the inoculum suspension to that of the standard, dip a sterile nontoxic cotton swab into the inoculum and remove excess inoculum by pressing and rotating the swab firmly against the side of the tube above the level of the liquid.
- Inoculate the dried surface of Mueller-Hinton agar plate that has been brought to room temperature by streaking the swab in three directions over the entire agar surface.
- Replace the lid of the dish. Allow 3–5 minutes but no longer than 15 minutes for surface of agar to dry before applying the antibiotic discs.

- Place the appropriate antibiotic discs on the surface of agar, using either sterile forceps or multidisc dispenser. After placement, press the disc on the surface of the medium to provide uniform contact. The disc must be evenly distributed on the agar so that they are not closer than 24 mm centre to centre. On a plate of 100 mm diameter, seven discs may be placed one in the centre and six in the periphery (Fig. 14.1). The plates are then incubated at 35–37° C for 16–18 hours.
- By using a caliper or transparent plastic ruler, the zones of complete growth inhibition around each of the discs are carefully measured. The diameter of the disc is included in this measurement. The zone size that is observed in a disc diffusion test has no meaning by itself. The interpretation of zone size is based on the interpretation chart (Table 14.1). Reference strains of *Staphylococcus aureus, Escherichia coli, Pseudomonas aeruginosa*, etc. should be tested each time a new batch of discs or agar is used.

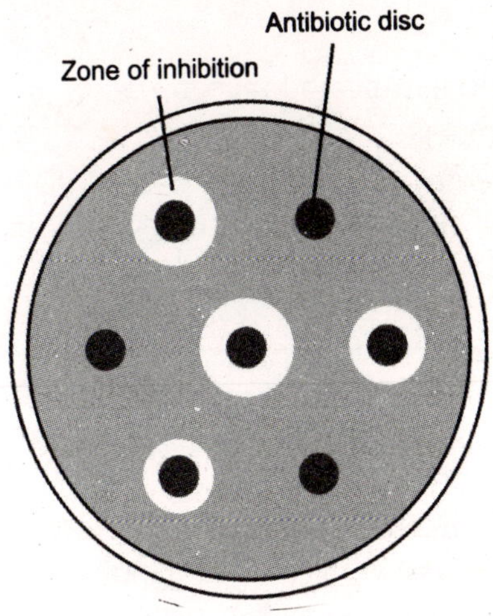

Fig. 14.1. Kirby-Bauer disc diffusion method.

Table 14.1. Interpretation chart of zone size in Kirby-Bauer disc diffusion method

Antimicrobial agent	*Diameter of zone of inhibition (mm)*		
	Resistant	*Moderately susceptible*	*Susceptible*
Benzyl penicillin	≤ 28	–	≥ 29
Ampicillin			
• Enterobacteriaceae	≤ 13	14–16	≥ 17
• Enterococci	≤ 16	–	≥ 17
• *Haemophilus* and *Moraxella* spp.	≤ 19	–	≥ 20
Cephalothin	≤ 14	15–17	≥ 18
Cefuroxime	≤ 14	15–17	≥ 18
Ceftazidime	≤ 14	15–17	≥ 18
Cefotaxime	≤ 14	15–22	≥ 23
Methicillin	≤ 9	10–13	≥ 14
Carbenicillin			
• *E. coli* and *Proteus* spp.	≤ 17	18–22	≥ 23
• *P. aeruginosa*	≤ 13	14–17	≥ 18
Gentamicin	≤ 12	–	≥ 13
Amikacin	≤ 14	15–16	≥ 17
Tobramycin	≤ 12	13–14	≥ 15
Erythromycin	≤ 13	14–17	≥ 18
Clindamycin	≤ 14	15–20	≥ 21
Tetracycline	≤ 14	15–18	≥ 19
Fusidic acid	≤ 14	15–18	≥ 19
Chloramphenicol	≤ 12	13–17	≥ 18
Colistin	≤ 8	9–10	≥ 11
Nalidixic acid	≤ 13	14–18	≥ 19
Nitrofurantoin	≤ 14	15–16	≥ 17
Trimethoprim	≤ 10	11–15	≥ 16
Trimethoprim/sulphamethoxazole	≤ 10	11–15	≥ 16
Ciprofloxacin	≤ 15	16–20	≥ 21
Piperacillin			
• Enterobacteriaceae	≤ 17	18–20	≥ 21
• *Pseudomonas*	≤ 14	15–17	≥ 18

Results

The Kirby-Bauer method recognizes three categories of susceptibility:

- *Susceptible* : An organism is called "susceptible" to a drug when the infection caused by it is likely to respond to treatment with this drug, at the recommended dosage.
- *Intermediate susceptible* : It is applicable to strains that are "moderately susceptible" to an antibiotic that can be used for treatment at a higher dosage because of its low toxity or because the antibiotic is concentrated at the focus of infection. The term also applies to those strains that are susceptible to a more toxic antibiotic that cannot be used at a higher dosage.
- *Resistant* : The organism does not respond to a given drug, irrespective of the dosage and the location of the infection.

Stokes disc diffusion method

- The Mueller-Hinton agar plate is divided into three parts. The test organism is inoculated on central one third and control on upper and lower thirds of the plate however, in modified stokes disc diffusion method, the test organism is inoculated in the upper and lower thirds and control on central one third.
- An uninoculated gap 2–3 mm wide should separate the test and control areas on which antibiotic discs are applied (Fig. 14.2).
- A maximum of six antibiotic discs can be placed on a single 100 mm diameter plate. The plates are then incubated at 35–37°C for 16–18 hours.

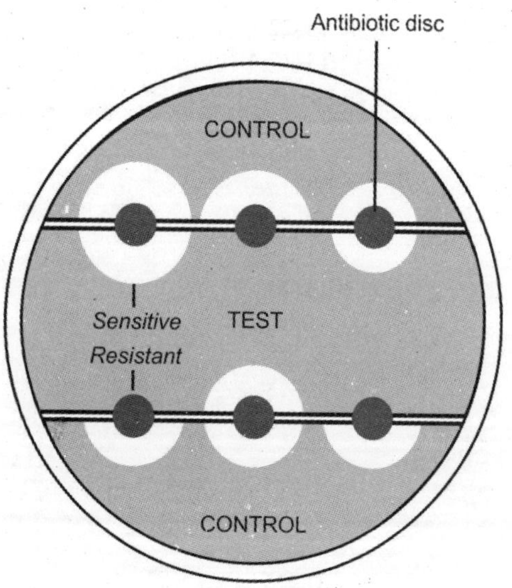

Fig. 14.2. Stokes disc diffusion test.

- Measure the zone size, i.e. the distance in mm from the edge of the disc to the zone edge, if that is obvious, if it is not, measure to the point of 80% or more inhibition of growth. However, if the test zones are obviously larger than the control or give no zone of inhibition at all, it is not necessary to perform any measurement.

Results

Zone size is interpreted as follows:

- *Sensitive* : The zone size is equal to, larger than or not more than 3 mm smaller than the control.
- *Intermediate* : The zone size of the test strain is at least 2 mm, but also at least 3 mm smaller than that of the control strain.
- *Resistant* : The zone size of the test strain is smaller than 2 mm.

Discussion

1. **What are the advantages of antimicrobial susceptibility testing?**
   It is used to guide the clinician in selecting the best antimicrobial agent and to accumulate epidemiological information on the resistance of microorganisms of public health importance.
2. **Which medium is preferred for antimicrobial sensitivity testing?**
   Mueller-Hinton agar
3. **How many antibiotic discs can be accommodated on a single 100 mm diameter plate?**
   Six or seven
4. **What are the advantages of Stokes disc diffusion method for antimicrobial susceptibility testing?**
   Reading of test strain is always taken in comparison to that of standard control. All blank discs (without antibiotics) can also be detected.
5. **Name various diffusion methods of antimicrobial sensitivity testing.**
   - Kirby-Bauer method
   - Stokes method

PART–2

Serology / Immunology

Contents

Practical 15

Venereal Disease Research Laboratory (VDRL) Test

Introduction

VDRL test is a nontreponemal test most widely employed for the diagnosis of syphilis. It is a simple and rapid test which requires only a small quantity of serum.

Principle

This is non-specific flocculation test. This test is performed as a slide test in which inactivated patient serum is mixed with a freshly prepared suspension of cardiolipin-lecithin-cholesterol antigen on a glass slide. The mixture is rotated, usually mechanically, for 7 minutes after which the flocculation (aggregation of antigen-antibody complexes in suspension) can be detected under a low power objective of a microscope. Reagin (antibodies that appear in syphilis) in the serum reacts with the VDRL antigen and forms floccules.

Requirements

- Serum
- Water-bath (56°C)
- VDRL rotator (180 r.p.m.)
- VDRL glass slides (7.5 × 5 cm) with 12 paraffin rings of approximately 15 mm diameter.
- Screw-capped bottle of 30 ml capacity with flat inner bottom surface
- Tuberculin syringe
- 18 gauge needle
- Pipettes 1.0, 5.0 ml
- VDRL kit: It contains (a) stock VDRL antigen in ampoules and, (b) buffered saline. It is necessary to prepare carefully a working VDRL antigen fresh before the test. Working VDRL antigen is stable at 0–4 °C only for 12 hours.

Method

Preparation of antigen

- Bring the buffered saline and antigen to room temperature.
- Pipette 0.4 ml of buffered saline into a 30 ml round bottomed screw-capped bottle.
- Add 0.5 ml of VDRL antigen with the help of a tuberculin syringe, drop by drop rapidly in 6 seconds while gently rotating the bottle in a circle of 5 cm diameter.
- Continue rotation of the bottle for 10 more seconds.
- Add 4.1 ml of buffered saline more.
- Replace the top of the bottle and shake it for 10 seconds.
- Allow it to stand for 15–30 minutes. The working antigen suspension may be used during whole working day.

Preparation of serum

Heat the serum in a water-bath at 56°C for 30 minutes to inactivate the complement and use within 4 hours. Reinactivate the serum for ten minutes if it cannot be processed within 4 hours.

Qualitative test

Carried on glass slides (7.5 × 5 cm), each with 12 paraffin rings.

- Pipette 50 μl of inactivated patient serum into the paraffin ring on the glass slide.

- Pipette 50 μl each of positive and negative control sera into other paraffin rings.
- Add one drop of working antigen suspension to each of these paraffin rings from a syringe delivering 60 drops in 1 ml.
- Mix with wooden sticks and rotate the slide for 4 minutes with hand on a flat surface in a circular manner in a diameter of about 5 cm or on a mechanical VDRL rotator set at about 180 r.p.m.
- Read the test results immediately under a low power objective of a microscope (Fig. 15.1). The antigen particles are seen as small fusiform needles which remain more or less evenly dispersed in case of non-reactive serum. Grouping of these particles into small or large clumps denotes the degree of reactivity and is interpreted as follows :

Medium and large clumps	Reactive
Small clumps	Weakly reactive
No clumps	Non-reactive

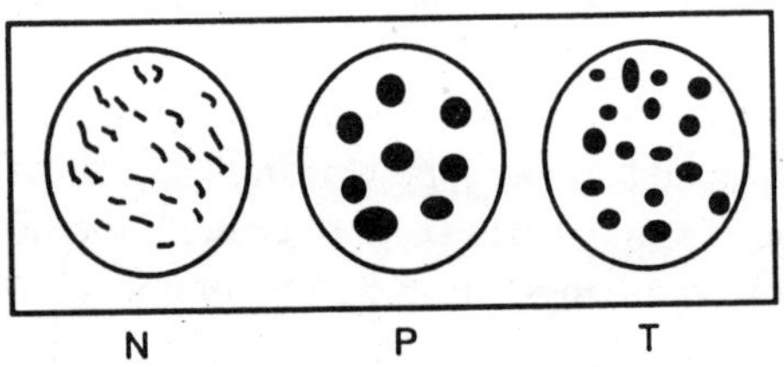

Fig. 15.1. VDRL slide test (N - negative control, P - positive control, T - test serum).

Any specimen giving a weak positive or positive reaction should then be tested quantitatively. It is performed with serial dilutions of patient serum. The highest dilution that can be classified as reactive is reported as the titre.

Quantitative VDRL test

- Place 6 test tubes in a rack.
- Add 200 μl of physiological saline in each tube.
- Add 200 μl of the patient serum in first tube and mix well. The dilution will be 1:2.
- Transfer 200 μl from the first up to sixth tube successively. The dilution will now be 1:2, 1:4, 1:8, 1:16, 1:32 and 1:64 respectively.
- Add 50 μl of each dilution to the respective paraffin rings. Include controls as in qualitative test.
- Add 1 drop of VDRL antigen i.e. 1/60 ml to each ring from a syringe.
- Rotate the slides on VDRL rotator adjusted at 180 r.p.m. for 4 minutes.

Reporting

Read the test immediately with 10X objective of light microscope. Report the titre as highest dilution of the serum that shows a reactive result. A titre of 1:16 and above for reaginic antibody is interpreted in favour of syphilis.

Interpretation

Since the VDRL antigen is non-specific in nature, the test is often reactive in several other clinical conditions characterized by production of reaginic antibody. These include lepromatous leprosy, malaria, relapsing fever, hepatitis, systemic lupus erythematosus, infectious mononucleosis and tropical eosinophilia and are collectively termed as **biological false positive reactions**. The diagnosis is confirmed by specific treponemal test and quantitative VDRL test.

Advantages

1. VDRL test is used as a screening test and is positive in approximately 70% of primary and 99% of secondary syphilis.
2. It becomes positive 10–14 days after the appearance of primary chancre.
3. Positive result in VDRL test usually indicates active infection, therefore, it can be used to monitor the efficacy of antibacterial therapy.
4. The VDRL test can be done on CSF and it is useful in diagnosis of neurosyphilis.

Disadvantages

1. Antigen has to be prepared fresh.
2. Heat-inactivation of sera is necessary to destroy a heat-labile inhibitory factor of IgM class.
3. Microscope is required to read the results.
4. Positive VDRL test should be confirmed by testing with a *Treponema pallidum* specific test.

Rapid plasma reagin (RPR) card test

RPR card test is a macroscopic nontreponemal flocculation test used for the detection and quantitation of antilipoidal antibodies (reagin).

Principle

Cardiolipin antigen is adsorbed on finely divided carbon particles and suspended in choline which blocks inhibitory factors in the serum thus eliminating the need to heat the serum before testing. The antigen is stabilized with EDTA, allowing it to be used for up to 6 months when stored at 4–10°C. This test is performed by mixing one drop of patient serum or plasma (50 μl), with a drop of this modified antigen (20 μl) on a disposable plastic card (12.5 × 7 cm in size with 10 clearly defined test areas) using a disposable stick. The card is then rocked gently to and fro for 8 minutes and observed under strong source of light. In a positive test, the flocculation of carbon particles (black aggregates) is visible with naked eye. Black aggregates may be deposited at the periphery of the liquid. In a negative case, there is a complete absence of black aggregates with a uniform greyish background.

Any specimen giving a positive reaction should then be tested quantitatively using doubling dilutions of serum.

Advantages

- Quick and easy to perform.
- Serum sample does not need to be heat-inactivated.
- Cards can be read macroscopically.

Disadvantage

It cannot be used to test cerebrospinal fluid.

Discussion

1. **Enumerate various nontreponemal tests or standard tests for syphilis (STS).**
    - Wasserman test
    - Kahn test
    - Venereal Disease Research Laboratory (VDRL) test
    - Rapid plasma reagin (RPR) test
2. **What is the principle of VDRL test?**
   Slide flocculation
3. **Which antigen is used in all nontreponemal tests?**
   The antigen used in nontreponemal tests is an alcoholic extract of beef-heart tissue (cardiolipin) to which lecithin and cholesterol are added.
4. **What is the principle of Kahn test and Wasserman test?**
   Tube flocculation test and complement fixation test respectively
5. **Why Kahn and Wasserman tests are not done now a days?**
   Because of the availability of simple and rapid tests e.g. VDRL and RPR tests.
6. **When does 'reagin' antibody develop in syphilitic patients?**
   Ten to 14 days after the appearance of primary chancre.
7. **Why serum sample is heat-inactivated for VDRL test?**
   Heat-inactivation of serum is necessary to destroy a heat-labile inhibitory factor of IgM class which may be present in both normal and syphilitic serum.
8. **What is the major advantage of VDRL over RPR test?**
   VDRL test can be used to test cerebrospinal fluid while RPR cannot be used.
9. **What do you mean by biological false positive (BFP) reaction?**
   Detection of antibodies against cardiolipin in the absence of *T. pallidum* infection is known as biological false positive reaction.
10. **How do you differentiate BFP from true positive?**
    In BFP cases, specific treponemal tests are negative and there is no history of present or past treponemal infection.
11. **How do you classify BFP reaction?**
    BFP may be divided into acute or transient and chronic BFP reactions:
    - *Acute or transient BFP reaction* : It develops shortly after an acute febrile infectious disease and disappears within a few weeks or months after the illness has subsided.
    - *Chronic BFP reaction* : It persists longer than six months. It may occur in a wide variety of infectious and non-infectious conditions associated with tissue damage.
12. **When do you get false negative VDRL test?**
    When the patient serum contains high titre of antibody (due to prozone phenomenon).
13. **What is the positivity rate of VDRL test in primary and secondary syphilis?**
    This test is positive in approximately 70% of primary and 99% of secondary syphilis. The titre of antibody may rise to 8 or 16 during primary syphilis and 16–128 during secondary syphilis.

14. **Which class of antibody present in patient serum causes suspension of cardiolipin antigen to flocculate?**

    IgM or IgG

15. **Why heat-inactivation of serum is not required in RPR test ?**

    In RPR test cardiolipin antigen is adsorbed on finely divided carbon particles and suspended in choline chloride which blocks inhibitory factors in the serum thus eliminating the need for heat-inactivation of the serum before testing.

16. **What precautions should be taken while testing CSF by VDRL test?**

    - CSF is not heat-inactivated.
    - VDRL antigen is sensitized with 10% saline.

Practical

16

Widal Test

Introduction

It is a tube agglutination test employed for the serological diagnosis of enteric fever, in which antibodies against *Salmonella* Typhi, *S.* Paratyphi A and B infections are detected in patient serum. Since two types of agglutinins are generated in the serum which react with 'O' and 'H' antigenic components of the salmonellae, a total of four antigen suspension namely TO, TH, AH and BH are employed in the test.

Principle

Tube agglutination test.

Requirements

- Widal rack
- Dreyer's tubes for 'H' agglutinins (conical bottom)
- Felix tubes for 'O' agglutinins (round bottom)
- Patient serum
- Antigen suspensions (commercially available or locally prepared)
- Physiological saline (0.85% sodium chloride)
- Pipettes
- Water-bath at 37°C

Procedure

1. Arrange four rows each containing 7 clean and dry Widal tubes in a Widal rack.
2. Mix 0.1 ml of the patient serum with 1.4 ml of the physiological saline to obtain a 1 in 15 dilution (master dilution).
3. Add 0.4 ml of saline from second to seventh tube with the help of a pipette.
4. Add 0.4 ml of freshly prepared 1 in 15 dilution of serum into the first two tubes of each row.
5. After mixing, transfer 0.4 ml from second tube onwards up to sixth tube and from sixth tube discard 0.4 ml.
6. Add 0.4 ml of respective antigen namely TO, TH, AH and BH in each row from first to seventh tube. The final dilution would be 1:30, 1:60, 1:120, 1:240, 1:480 and 1:960 in the first six tubes respectively, while the last tube would serve as negative control (Fig. 16.1).
7. Incubate the tubes at 37°C in a water-bath for 4 hours and read after overnight refrigeration at 4°C.

Results

'H' agglutination leads to the formation of loose and cotton-woolly clumps, while 'O' agglutination appears as a disc-like granular deposit at the bottom of the tube. Control tube (Felix) shows a compact deposit. The highest dilution of the serum showing agglutination indicates the titre of the antibody.

Interpretation

1) Agglutinins usually appear by seventh to tenth day of illness in enteric fever, so that a negative result at an early stage is inconclusive. The titre then increases steadily till the third or fourth week, after which it declines gradually.

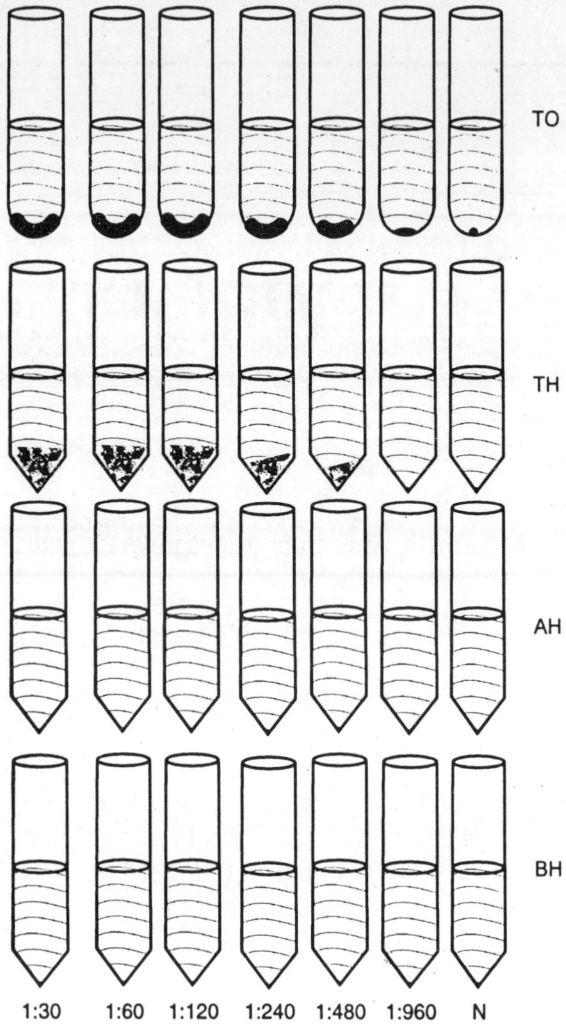

Fig. 16.1. Widal test (N-negative control).

2) Demonstration of rising titre, e.g. four-fold or greater, between tests made in the first and third weeks is highly significant. However, if the first sample is taken late in the disease, a rise may not be demonstrable. Instead a fall in titre may be seen in some cases.
3) Though it is generally stated that titres of 1:100 or more for O agglutinins and 1:200 or more for H agglutinins are significant, the results in a single test by no means prove the presence of enteric fever nor negative results its absence.
4) Serum from individuals immunized with TAB vaccine may show high titres of antibodies to *S.* Typhi, *S.* Paratyphi A and *S.* Paratyphi B. However, if a marked rise of titre to one serotype is observed, the results may be regarded as diagnostically significant. H agglutinins tend to persist for many months after vaccination but O agglutinins tend to disappear sooner i.e. within 6 months. Therefore, rise in O agglutinins indicate recent infection.
5) For determining the serotype of infecting organism, H agglutinin is more reliable than O agglutinin because the different serotypes have some O antigens in common. Moreover, O antigens are also widely distributed among other enterobacteria.
6) Persons who had past enteric infection or who have been vaccinated may develop **anamnestic** response during an unrelated fever like malaria, influenza, etc. The anamnestic response shows only a transient rise, in titre, while in enteric fever the rise is sustained.
7) Test suspensions of bacteria may contain non-specific antigens such as fimbrial antigens which may produce false positive results.
8) In many healthy individuals, the Widal reaction may be positive in the carrier state. This can be recognized by positive reaction with 'Vi' agglutinins in a titre of $\geq$ 1:10.

Discussion

1. **What is the principle of Widal test?**
   Tube agglutination
2. **What are the uses of Widal test?**
   - This is an important diagnostic test for quantitative estimation of antibodies in enteric fever.
   - Causative salmonellae can be diagnosed, i.e. *S.* Typhi, *S.* Paratyphi A, *S.* Paratyphi B and *S.* Paratyphi C.
   - Declining titre with antibiotics indicates patient is responding to treatment.
   - Progression of disease can be diagnosed with increasing antibody titre.
3. **Why Paratyphi 'O' antigen (Paratyphi A, Paratyphi B) is not employed in Widal test?**
   Because they cross react with *Salmonella* Typhi 'O' antigen due to sharing by them of factor 12.
4. **Enumerate various antigens of salmonellae.**
   - Flagellar (H) antigens
   - Somatic (O) antigens
   - Fimbrial (F) antigens
   - Surface (Vi, M) antigens
5. **Which of the somatic or flagellar antigens is more antigenic?**
   Flagellar antigen is more antigenic.

6. **Which antigen is heat-labile?**
'H' (flagellar) antigen

7. **Which standard strain of *S.* Typhi is used for preparation of O antigen?**
For the preparation of O antigen *S.* Typhi 901 strain is used.

8. **When do agglutinins appear during the course of enteric fever?**
Agglutinins usually appear by seventh to tenth day of enteric fever.

9. **In which condition all tubes show agglutination?**
In TAB vaccinated person

10. **Which agglutinins indicate recent infection?**
Rise in O agglutinins

11. **Which agglutinins disappear first after infection?**
'O' agglutinins. They tend to disappear within 6 months, while 'H' agglutinins tend to persist for nearly 2 years.

12. **How do you differentiate anamnestic reaction from true enteric fever?**
In both conditions agglutinins against 'O' and 'H' antigens are raised in the blood. However, the rise is transient in anamnestic reaction whereas in enteric fever, it is sustained.

13. **In which conditions Widal test may be negative in case of enteric fever?**
    - Patient on antibiotic treatment
    - When Widal test is done in first week.

14. **What are the other serological methods to detect antibodies in patient serum in enteric fever?**
    - Indirect haemagglutination test
    - Counterimmunoelectrophoresis
    - ELISA/solid-phase RIA

15. **Which agglutinin has been claimed to indicate the carrier state?**
Vi agglutinins ≥ 1:10

16. **How would you diagnose a carrier of *Salmonella*?**
    - Demonstration of Vi agglutinins (≥ 1: 10)
    - Faecal culture
    - Bile culture
    - Urine culture

17. **How much titre is diagnostic in Widal test?**
Rising titres in paired sera is diagnostic. In a single test ≥ 1:100 titre of 'O' and ≥ 1:200 titre of 'H' is significant.

18. **In which conditions result of Widal test is doubtful?**
    - Past exposure to infection
    - Previous immunization with TAB vaccine
    - Early antibiotic treatment

19. **Which cancer may be seen in chronic typhoid carriers?**
Hepatobiliary cancer

20. **Which *Salmonella* spp. is more associated with chronic carriers?**
Salmonella Typhi

21. **Where do the salmonellae reside in a carrier?**
Salmonellae reside in gall bladder, biliary tract and rarely in intestine and urinary tract.

22. **Why do you collect repeated samples of faeces or bile to diagnose a chronic carrier of *Salmonella*?**
Because there is intermittent shedding of the organisms.

23. **What is the main advantage of detection of carriers?**
This helps in screening food handlers and cooks. So detection of carriers is important for epidemiological and public health purposes.

24. **What is the treatment of choice for chronic carriers?**
    - Antibiotics (ampicillin, amoxycillin and co-trimoxazole)
    - Cholecystectomy

Practical 17

Complement Fixation Test

Introduction

The term complement (C) is applied to a system of components present in the serum of man and animals. It consists of nine different proteins denoted C_1–C_9, some of which are heat-labile and are destroyed by heating at 56°C for 30 minutes. Serum deprived of C activity is said to be inactivated. Complement takes part in many immunological reactions and gets adsorbed during the combination of antigen (Ag) and antibody without any visible effect. This property of antigen and antibody complex to fix the complement is used in complement fixation test (CFT) for the identification of specific antibodies and antigens. The haemolytic system containing sheep erythrocytes and its corresponding antibody (amboceptor) is used as an indicator which shows the utilization or availability of the complement.

Principle

Complement lyses antibody-coated red cells. If the complement is fixed then there will be no lysis of erythrocytes, thus denoting a positive test. If the complement is available then there will be haemolysis which is a property of complement, thus denoting a negative test.

Requirements

- Patient serum (inactivated by heating in water-bath at 56°C for 30 minutes)
- Physiological saline
- Complement (pooled guinea-pig serum)
- Sheep RBCs.
- Amboceptor (antisheep red cell antibody)
- Centrifuge machine
- Antigen (soluble or particulate)
- Microtitre plate and micropipettes

Procedure

The procedure is carried out in two stages:

1. In stage1, test serum (for the detection of antibody) and the antigen are mixed in the presence of carefully measured amount of complement and then incubated at 37°C for 1 hour. If the test serum contains antibody then antigen-antibody complexes are formed and complement gets fixed on it.
2. In stage 2, indicator system, antibody-coated sheep red cells, is added to determine whether the complement has been fixed in stage 1 reaction or not. If the complement is taken up during stage 1 reaction then it will not be available to lyse the red cells, while a negative test, with unused complement, is shown by lysis of the red cells (Fig. 17.1).

Interpretation

Ag	Ag
+	+
Patient serum containing Ab	Patient serum containing no Ab
+	+
C	C
+	+
Haemolytic system	Haemolytic system
↓	↓
No haemolysis (Test positive)	Haemolysis (Test negative)

Fig. 17.1. Complement fixation test.

Uses

1) This is a very sensitive test and can detect as little as 0.04 μg of antibody and 0.1 μg of antigen.
2) Wassermann reaction and Reiter protein complement fixation test (RPCFT) for serodiagnosis of syphilis are based on this test.
3) CFT is useful for identification of bacterial, viral, fungal, chlamydial and parasitic antigen.

Discussion

1. **Why do you heat serum at 56°C for 30 minutes for CFT?**
   To inactivate complement present in the serum. It also inactivates certain non-specific factors which are likely to interfere with antigen-antibody reaction.
2. **What is the principle of Wassermann reaction?**
   Complement fixation test
3. **Which test is more specific (Wassermann or VDRL)?**
   Wassermann
4. **What do you mean by amboceptor?**
   Rabbit antibody to sheep red cells prepared by inoculating sheep erythrocytes into rabbit under standard immunization protocol, is known as amboceptor.
5. **Name pathways of complement activation.**
   Classical pathway and alternative pathway
6. **Which classes of immunoglobulins are involved in classical pathway?**
   IgG (IgG3,1,2) and IgM
7. **Which class of immunoglobulin can activate alternative pathway of complement activation?**
   IgA
8. **Name the factors which can activate alternative pathway of complement activation.**
   - Bacterial endotoxin
   - Rabbit RBCs
   - Snake venom proteins
   - Nephritic factor
   - Yeast cell wall
9. **Which subclass of IgG cannot fix complement?**
   IgG4
10. **Where is the complement binding site located in the immunoglobulin?**
    Complement binding site is located on the Fc piece of the immunoglobulin molecule (C_H2 domain on IgG and C_H4 on IgM).
11. **What happens if there is complement deficiency in the serum?**
    It leads to recurrent bacterial and fungal infections. Collagen diseases also occur in complement deficiency.

Practical 18

Enzyme Immunoassay (EIA)

Introduction

The term enzyme immunoassay (EIA) includes all assays based on the measurement of enzyme-labelled antigen, hapten or antibody. EIAs are of two basic types: homogeneous and heterogeneous. In homogeneous EIA, there is no need to separate the bound and free fractions so that the test can be completed in one step, with all reagents added simultaneously. Heterogeneous EIA requires the separation of the free and bound fractions either by centrifugation or by absorption on solid surface and washing. It is, therefore, a multistep procedure, with reagents added sequentially. The major type of heterogeneous EIA is enzyme-linked immunosorbent assay (ELISA).

ELISA

ELISA is a highly sensitive and specific test used for the detection of a variety of antigens and antibodies of microbial and human origin. ELISA test is classified into 3 types depending upon the source of antigen used in the test proper. They are:

1) first generation ELISA,
2) second generation ELISA and,
3) third generation ELISA.

Principle

Antigen or antibody is adsorbed on the solid-phase which may be polystyrene or polyvinyl microtitre plates. Test serum with antigen or antibody is added and incubated at 37°C for 2 hours for formation of antigen-antibody complex and unbound components are finally removed by washing. The amount of bound fraction is subsequently measured by addition of enzyme-linked anti-human globulin or specific antibody and an appropriate substrate to produce colour and products detected by the ELISA reader.

Requirements

- Patient serum
- Diagnostic kit
  - Microtitre plate
  - Enzyme conjugate (peroxidase-labelled purified antigen)
  - Buffered substrate (contains H_2O_2).
  - Chromogen solution (tetramethylbenzidine in dimethyl sulfoxide)
  - Stopping solution (sulphuric acid)
  - Washing solution
  - Sample diluent
  - Negative control
  - Positive control
  - Cut-off serum
  - Conjugate diluent
  - Diluents for reagents and specimen
- Microplate—ELISA reader

Procedure

1. Add appropriate volume of diluent in each well.
2. Add appropriate volume of test serum and equal volume of positive and negative controls into the respective wells of microtitre plate.
3. Cover the plate with adhesive film and incubate at 37°C for specified time.
4. Aspirate the contents and wash the wells four times by using working wash solution. Now add appro-

priate volume of the conjugate. Mix well and incubate at 37°C for specified time.
5. Aspirate the contents and wash the wells five times by using wash solution.
6. Add appropriate volume of buffered substrate and chromogen solutions. Incubate at 37°C for specified time.
7. Add stop solution and read absorbance bichromatically at 450 nm and 660 nm by using a microplate reader.

Uses

ELISA kits have been developed for detecting:

- HIV-1 and HIV-2 antigens and antibody.
- *Entamoeba histolytica* antigens in faeces.
- *Toxoplasma* antigens in patient serum.
- *Haemophilus influenzae* antigens in spinal fluid.
- β-haemolytic streptococcal antigens in spinal fluid.
- Hepatitis A virus in stools.
- Respiratory syncytial virus in pharyngeal secretions.
- Adenovirus antigens in nasopharyngeal specimens.
- Labile enterotoxin of *Escherichia coli* in stools.
- Hepatitis B surface antigen and its antibody.
- Cytomegalovirus antigen.
- Rubella IgG and IgM.
- *Mycobacterium tuberculosis* IgA.
- Thyroid hormones T_3, T_4 and TSH.

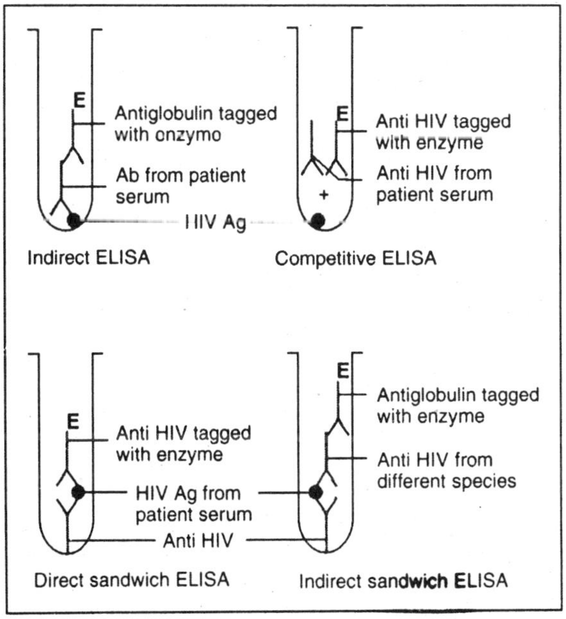

Fig. 18.1. ELISA.

Discussion

1. **What do you mean by first, second and third generation ELISA?**
   - *First generation ELISA*: Here the antigen is prepared by propagating viruses in mammalian cell line. It is coated on microwell plates after disrupting and inactivating the viral concentrate.
   - *Second generation ELISA*: Here the antigen is prepared either by bacterial recombinant DNA technology or proteins which corresponds to viral component.
   - *Third generation ELISA*: Here the synthetic peptides are used as antigen source and they generally correspond to viral antigenic epitopes.
2. **What do you mean by immunosorbent in term ELISA?**

   An absorbing material specific for one of the components of the reaction, the antigen or antibody.
3. **Name different types of ELISA.**
   - Indirect ELISA
   - Competitive ELISA
   - Sandwich ELISA(direct and indirect)

   The diagrammatic represenatation of these is given in Fig. 18.1.
4. **What do you mean by indirect ELISA?**

   This is used for the detection of antibody and, therefore, the solid-phase is conjugated with antigen.
5. **Describe briefly competitive ELISA.**

   This method can be used for detection of antigen or antibody. For the detection of antibodies, solid-phase is coated with antigen. Test sample and enzyme-labelled specific antibody conjugate are added at the same time for specific period. During incubation there is competition between antibodies of patient serum and specific antibody conjugate for sharing of antigen. Intense colour suggests the binding of specific antibody conjugate and hence a non-reactive reaction, while lack of colour indicates binding of patient serum antibodies and hence a reactive reaction.
6. **How many types of sandwich ELISA are known to you?**

   Two types:
   - Single antibody or direct sandwich ELISA
   - Double antibody or indirect sandwich ELISA

7. **What is the difference between EIA and radioimmunoassay (RIA)?**

   Both these tests are based on the same principle. The key difference is that for enzyme immunoassays the antigen or antibody is conjugated to an enzyme rather than a radioactive isotope.

8. **What is the function of this enzyme?**

   Enzyme converts a colourless substrate into a coloured one.

9. **Which enzymes are commonly used in this test?**
   - Horseradish peroxidase
   - Alkaline phosphatase

10. **What are the advantages of ELISA test?**
    - Highly sensitive
    - Safe and economical
    - Simple instrumentation required
    - Many tests can be performed at the same time.

PART–3

Parasitology

Contents

Practical 19

Collection and Preservation of Stool Specimen

Introduction

Stool or faeces sample is the most common specimen used for the diagnosis of intestinal parasitic infections. Depending on the nature of the parasite the microscopic observations include the identification of cysts, ova, trophozoites, larvae or portions of the adult structure. The ability to detect and identify human parasite is directly linked to the quality of the clinical specimen.

Collection of the specimen

1. Specimen should be collected in a wide-mouthed clean container without contamination with urine, water or disinfectants.
2. The collection of three faecal specimens usually suffice to make the diagnosis of intestinal parasitic diseases, two obtained on successive days during normal bowel movement and a third after magnesium sulphate purge. A total of six specimens, collected on successive days, may be required if intestinal amoebiasis or giardiasis is suspected.
3. The specimen should be free of oil and other nonfaecal substances such as barium or bismuth. Patients who have received a barium enema may not excrete organisms in their stool for at least 1 week following barium enema, therefore, stool examination must be delayed for at least 1 week following the enema.
4. Cathartics with an oil base should be avoided because oils retard motility of trophozoites and distort the morphology of the parasite.
5. The specimen should be properly labelled with patient's name, age, sex and date of collection.
6. Liquid stool specimens should be examined within 30 minutes after collection or semiformed stool within 60 minutes to detect motile trophozoites, particularly in suspected infections with *Entamoeba histolytica* and *Giardia lamblia.* Formed stools, in which trophozoites are not expected, may be examined up to 24 hours after passage.
7. Specimen should not be kept at the warm temperature and drying of the specimen should be prevented.

Preservation of specimen

Preservation of stool helps in maintaining morphology of protozoan parasites and preventing further development of some helminthic eggs and larvae. Since the preservatives kill parasites, therefore, characteristic motility of trophozoites cannot be seen.

Discussion

1. **Which type of container is used for collecting faecal samples?**
   Samples should be collected in a wide-mouthed clean container.
2. **Why contamination with urine and water should be avoided while collecting faecal sample?**
   Because urine can destroy motile trophozoites and water may contain free-living organisms, which may be mistaken for human parasites.
3. **Enumerate some medications which interfere in the detection of parasites.**
   - Bismuth
   - Mineral oil
   - Kaolin

- Barium sulphate
- Certain antibiotics: tetracyclines, sulphonamides
- Anti-diarrhoeal agents

4. **How many faecal specimens are sufficient to make the diagnosis of intestinal parasitic diseases?**

   Three faecal specimens usually suffice to make the diagnosis of intestinal parasitic diseases. However, if intestinal amoebiasis or giardiasis is suspected then a total of six specimens collected on successive days, may be required.

5. **When should you examine the faecal specimens after collection?**

   The liquid stool specimens should be examined immediately within 30 minutes of passage and the semi-formed and soft specimens within 60 minutes of passage.

6. **How many faecal specimens are collected after treatment?**

   Three specimens (same as for diagnosis)

7. **What are the advantages of preservation of faecal specimens?**

   Preservation of stool helps in:
   - Maintaining morphology of protozoan parasites.
   - Preventing further development of some helminthic eggs and larvae.

8. **Enumerate the commonly used preservatives.**
   - Formalin solution
   - Polyvinyl alcohol (PVA)
   - Merthiolate-iodine-formalin solution (MIF)
   - Schaudinn's solution
   - Sodium acetate acetic acid-formalin fixative (SAF)

Practical 20

Examination of Stool

Examination of stool consists of macroscopic and microscopic examination.

I. Macroscopic examination

(1) **Consistency**: It may indicate types of organisms present. Trophozoites are usually found in soft or liquid specimens and cysts are found in semisolid or solid specimens.

Consistency	*Reasons*
(a) Well formed	Normal
(b) Hard	Constipation
(c) Watery	Bacterial infection, purgative
(d) Rice water stools	Cholera
(e) Pale, bulky and frothy	Steatorrhea
(f) Flattened and ribbon like	Obstruction in the lumen of bowel
(g) Semi-solid	Mild diarrhoea, after taking laxative, digestive upset.

(2) **Adult worms**: Following adult worms may be present in the stool:
Round worm
Pin worm
Hook worm
Tape worm

(3) **Colour**: Normal colour of the stool is light to dark brown (due to the presence of bile pigments).

Abnormal colour	*Reasons*
(a) Black	Bleeding in the upper gastrointestinal tract (GIT), iron intake.
(b) Bright red	Bleeding at the lower GIT level.
(c) Blood and mucus	Dysentery.
(d) Clay coloured	Obstruction to the flow of bile to intestine.
(e) White or light tan	After barium meal.

II. Microscopic examination

Intestinal protozoa, and eggs and larvae of helminths can be detected and identified by microscopic examination of the stool by :

1. Direct smear
2. Smear after concentration
3. Permanent stained smear.

1. Direct smear

Saline wet mount

Saline wet mount is made by mixing a small quantity (about 2 mg) of faeces in a drop of saline placed on a clean glass slide. Remove any gross fibres or particles and cover with a cover-slip. Avoid air bubble by drawing one edge of cover-slip slightly into the suspension and lowering it almost to the slide before letting it fall. The mount should be just thick enough that newspaper print can be read through the slide. The smear is then examined under microscope. Begin at one corner of the smear and systematically examine successive adjacent swaths (Fig. 20.1) with the low power of the microscope. When a parasite-like object comes into view, it should be more closely examined and identified under high power. Saline wet mount is used for the detection of trophozoites and cysts of protozoa and eggs and larvae of helminths. It is particularly useful for detection of live motile trophozoites of *Entamoeba histolytica, Giardia lamblia* and *Balantidium coli.*

Iodine wet mount

Stool is emulsified in a drop of five times diluted solution of Lugol's iodine on a clean glass slide, covered with a clean cover-slip and examined under microscope as above. Both saline and iodine wet mounts may be prepared on the same slide (Fig. 20.1). For the preparation of Lugol's iodine, 10 g of potassium iodide is dissolved in 100 ml distilled water and 5 g of iodine crystals are then added slowly. The solution is filtered and kept in a stoppered bottle of amber colour. It should be prepared every two weeks.

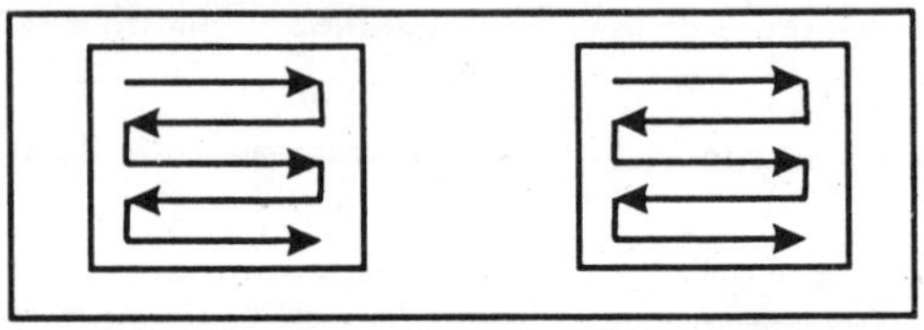

Fig. 20.1. Examination of a faecal smear (saline and iodine mount).

Iodine wet mount is used for the study of the nuclear character of cysts and trophozoites for the identification of the species. However, iodine immobilizes trophozoites. Iodine stained cysts of *E. histolytica* show pale refractile nuclei, yellowish cytoplasm and brown glycogen mass. The chromidial bars do not stain with iodine. Helminthic eggs and larvae are readily identified without stain, but the iodine stain can be used advantageously in the examination of larvae as it immobilizes and kills them and stain some parts differentially.

(2) Smear after concentration

The concentration of stool allows the detection of small number of parasites present in stool specimens. This procedure allows the increased recovery of eggs and larvae of helminths and cysts of protozoa. Trophozoites of the protozoa are destroyed during the concentration procedure. Two commonly used methods are :

- Floatation techniques
- Sedimentation techniques

Both these methods are designed to separate intestinal protozoa and helminthic eggs from excess of faecal debris by their differences in the specific gravity.

Floatation techniques

Floatation involves suspending the specimen in a medium of greater density than that of the helminthic eggs and protozoan cysts. The eggs and cysts float to the top and are collected by placing a glass slide on the surface of the meniscus at the top of the tube. Following floatation techniques can be used:

- Saturated salt floatation technique
- Zinc sulphate centrifugal floatation technique.

Sedimentation techniques

Concentration of intestinal parasites by sedimentation techniques, using either gravity or centrifugation, leads to a good recovery of cysts of protozoa and eggs of helminths. Cysts and eggs of parasites settle and are concentrated at the bottom because they have greater density than the suspending medium.

Following are the commonly used sedimentation techniques:

- Simple sedimentation
- Formalin-ether sedimentation

Discussion

1. **Which iodine solution should be used for iodine staining?**

   Weak iodine solution should be used. Gram's iodine is unsuitable, but Lugol's or D'Antoni's iodine solutions can be used.

2. **Why weak iodine solution should be used for iodine staining?**

   Because too strong solution of iodine can obscure the details of parasite.

3. **What is the appearance of *Entamoeba histolytica* cysts on iodine staining?**

   Body of the parasite : Yellow to light brown, and the nucleus is clearly seen with a central karyosome
   Cytoplasm : Smooth and hyaline
   Glycogen mass : Brown
   Chromatoid bars : Not stained

4. **Enumerate methods of stool concentration.**
   - Floatation techniques
   - Sedimentation techiniques

5. **Enumerate commonly used floatation techniques.**
   - Saturated salt floatation
   - Zinc sulphate centrifugal floatation

6. **Enumerate larvae and eggs which do not float in saturated salt solution.**
   - Unfertilized eggs of *Ascaris lumbricoides*
   - Eggs of *Taenia solium, T. saginata* and all intestinal flukes
   - *Strongyloides stercoralis* larvae

7. **Enumerate parasites which are stained by modified acid-fast stain.**
   - *Cryptosporidium parvum*
   - *Cyclospora* spp.
   - *Isospora belli*

8. **What is the concentration of sulphuric acid used in modified acid-fast technique?**

   Five per cent

9. **What is the colour of oocysts in faecal smears stained with modified acid-fast technique?**

   Oocysts stain red against green background.

10. **Name the swab used for the diagnosis of *Enterobius vermicularis* infection.**

    NIH swab

11. **What is Charcot Leyden crystal?**

    This is a breakdown product of granules of eosinophils.

12. **Which consistency of stool is best for examination of trophozoites?**

    Trophozoites are best seen in liquid stool.

13. **Enumerate the differences between a macrophage and trophozoite of *E. histolytica.***

Features	Trophozoite of *E. histolytica*	Macrophage
• Average size	20 µm	30–60 µm may be 5–10 µm
• Ratio of nuclear material to cytoplasm	1:10–1:12	1:4–1:6
• Cytoplasm	May contain red blood cells and some debris, and polymorphonuclear leucocytes.	Uaually contains ingested debris, red blood cells and polymorphonuclear leucocytes.
• Nucleus	One nucleus. It is round with central karyosome and peripheral fine chromatin granules.	One large nucleus that may be irregular.

Practical

21

Identification of Faecal Eggs

Ascaris lumbricoides (Round worm)

Fertilized eggs

The fertilized eggs are round or oval in shape and measure 60–75 μm in length and 40–50 μm in breadth. They are bile-stained and brown in colour. They are surrounded by a thick, transparent shell, consisting of a relatively nonpermeable innermost lipoidal vitelline membrane; a thick transparent middle layer and an outermost coarsely mammillated albuminoid layer (Colour Plate IV, Fig. 11). Outer mammillated coat is sometimes lost. Such eggs are called decorticated eggs. They contain a large conspicuous unsegmented ovum with a clear crescentic area at each pole. Fertilized eggs float in saturated solution of common salt.

Unfertilized eggs

In the absence of a male worm, the female produces unfertilized (infertile) eggs. These are narrower and longer and measure 90 μm in length and 55 μm in breadth. They are bile-stained and brown in colour. They have a small atrophied ovum and a thin shell within an irregular coating of albumin. The innermost lipoidal vitelline membrane of the shell is absent (Colour Plate IV, Fig. 12). The unfertilized eggs are heaviest of all the helminthic eggs, therefore, they do not float in saturated solution of common salt.

Enterobius vermicularis (Pin worm/thread worm)

The eggs are colourless, not bile-stained and flattened on one side (planoconvex). They measure 60 μm in length and 30 μm in width. They are surrounded by a thin, smooth, transparent shell and usually contain fully developed larvae (Colour Plate IV, Fig. 13). They float in saturated solution of common salt.

Ancylostoma duodenale and Necator americanus (Hook worm)

Eggs are oval or elliptical measuring 60 μm in length and 40 μm in width. They are colourless (not bile-stained) and are surrounded by a thin transparent hyaline shell. They possess a segmented ovum with usually four blastomeres (Colour Plate IV, Fig. 14). There is a clear space between the segmented ovum and the egg shell. The eggs float in saturated salt solution.

Trichuris trichiura (Whip worm)

The eggs are barrel-shaped with a mucous plug at each pole. Shell is yellow to brown(bile-stained) and plugs are colourless. They measure 50–54 μm × 22–23 μm in size (Colour Plate IV, Fig. 15). They float in saturated solution of common salt. When freshly passed, they contain unsegmented ova and are not infective to man.

Taenia saginata and Taenia solium (Beef tapeworm and pork tapeworm)

Eggs of both these species are indistinguishable. They are spherical, brown in colour (bile-stained) and measure 31–43 μm in diameter. They are surrounded by embryophore which is brown, thick-walled and radially striated. Outside this may be present thin transparent shell which represents the remnant of yolk mass. Inside the embryophore is present hexacanth embryo (oncosphere) with three pairs of hooklets (Colour Plate IV, Fig. 16). It does not float in saturated solution of common salt. The eggs of *T.solium* are infective to pig and also to man, while those of *T. saginata* are infective only to cattle.

Hymenolepis nana (The dwarf tapeworm)

Egg is spherical or oval, hyaline, 35–40 μm in diameter. It has a smooth, thin and colourless outer shell and an inner membrane (embryophore), containing a hexacanth embryo (oncosphere). The space between two membranes is filled with yolk granules and 4–8 polar filaments emanating from polar thickenings at either end of embryophore. It is non-bile-stained and floats in saturated solution of common salt (Colour Plate IV, Fig. 17).

Discussion

1. **Enumerate parasites whose eggs do not float in saturated salt solution.**
   - Unfertilized eggs of *A. lumbricoides*
   - *D. latum*
   - *Taenia solium* and *Taenia saginata*
   - Eggs of all intestinal flukes
2. **Enumerate parasites whose eggs are non-bile-stained.**
   - *Ancylostoma duodenale*
   - *Necator americanus*
   - *Hymenolepis nana*
3. **Name one ovo-viviparous nematode.**
   Strongyloides stercoralis
4. **Name one parasite whose eggs are detected in urine.**
   Schistosoma haematobium
5. **Name one parasite whose egg is planoconvex.**
   E. vermicularis
6. **Eggs of which parasites are considered heaviest of all the helminthic eggs?**
   Unfertilized eggs of *A. lumbricoides*
7. **What do you mean by decorticated eggs of *A. lumbricoides?***
   If outermost mammillated albuminoid layer of eggs is lost, then they are known as decorticated eggs.
8. **Name one parasite whose eggs can be detected in sputum.**
   Paragonimus westermani

Practical 22

Identification of Faecal Trophozoites, Cysts and Oocysts

Entamoeba histolytica

Trophozoite

It measures 10–60 μm (average 20–30 μm) in diameter. The cytoplasm of the trophozoite can be divided into a clear outer ectoplasm and an inner finely granular endoplasm in which red blood cells, leucocytes and tissue debris are found within the food vacuoles. Red blood cells may, however, be absent if infection is confined to the gut lumen. Trophozoites are motile. Movement results from long finger-like pseudopodial extensions of ectoplasm into which endoplasm flows. Trophozoite is the only form present in the tissues. It usually appears only in diarrhoeic faeces in active cases and survives only for a few hours. Nucleus is spherical in shape varying in size from 4–6 μm in diameter. In stained preparations it shows a central dot-like karyosome which is surrounded by a clear halo. The nuclear membrane is delicate and is lined by a single layer of fine chromatin granules. The space between the karyosome and the nuclear membrane is traversed by linin network (achromatic fibrils) having spoke-like radial arrangement (Fig. 22.1).

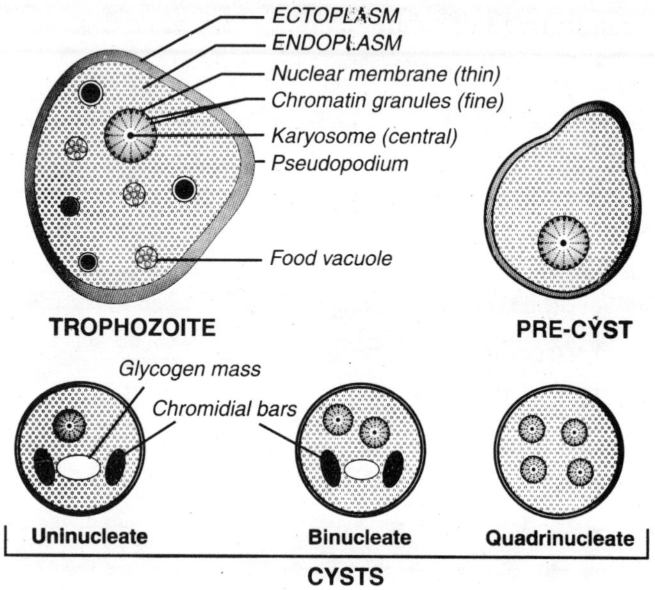

Fig. 22.1. Morphological forms of *Entamoeba histolytica*.

Cyst

It is spherical, 10–15 μm in diameter. It is surrounded by a thick chitinous wall which makes it highly resistant to the gastric acid, adverse environmental conditions and the chlorine concentration found in potable water. It starts as a uninucleate body, but later the nucleus divides to form two and then four nuclei (Fig. 22.1). Uninucleate and binucleate cysts in addition also possess a glycogen mass, which stains brown with iodine, and 1–4 chromidial or chromatoid bars (Colour Plate IV, Fig. 18). These do not stain with iodine but appear as refractile oblong bars with rounded ends in normal saline preparations. With iron-haematoxylin stain they stain black in colour.

Entamoeba coli

Trophozoite

It measures 20–50 μm in diameter. The cytoplasm is not defined and contain bacteria and cellular debris but never red blood cells (Fig. 22.2). Trophozoites are motile. They extend pseudopodia in multiple planes and "wander" aimlessly in one direction then the other. Nucleus shows eccen-

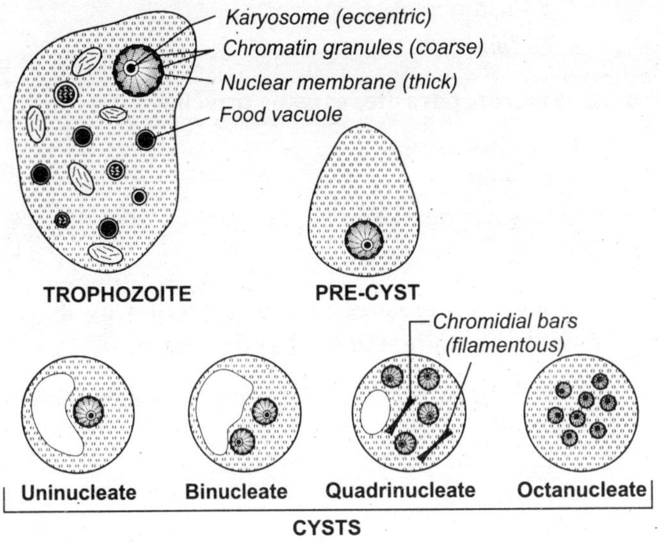

Fig. 22.2. Morphological forms of *Entamoeba coli.*

tric karyosome. The nuclear membrane is thick and is lined by coarse chromatin granules. Nucleus is visible in ustained preparation.

Cyst

It is spherical and 15–20 μm in diameter (Fig. 22.2 and Colour Plate IV, Fig. 19). It contain 1–8 nuclei and chromidial bars are filamentous. It lives freely in the lumen of large intestine of man and is nonpathogenic.

Giardia lamblia

Trophozoite

It is pear-shaped with rounded anterior and pointed posterior end (Fig. 22.3 and Colour Plate IV, Fig. 21). It measures 10–20 μm in length and 5–15 μm in width. The dorsal surface is convex while on the ventral surface it has a shallow posteriorly notched concavity (sucking disc) that embraces anterior half of the organism. It acts as an organelle of attachment. It is bilaterally symmetrical and has one pair of nuclei, one on each side of the midline, one pair of axostyles, one pair of parabasal bodies present on the axostyles, four pairs of flagella and probably four pairs of blepharoplasts from which the flagella arise.

Cyst

Mature cyst is oval in shape and measures 11–14 μm × 7–10 μm in size. It has two pairs of nuclei which may remain clustered at one end or lie in pairs at opposite ends. The remains of the flagella and margins of the sucking disc may be seen inside the cytoplasm of the cyst (Fig. 22.3 and Colour Plate IV, Fig. 22).

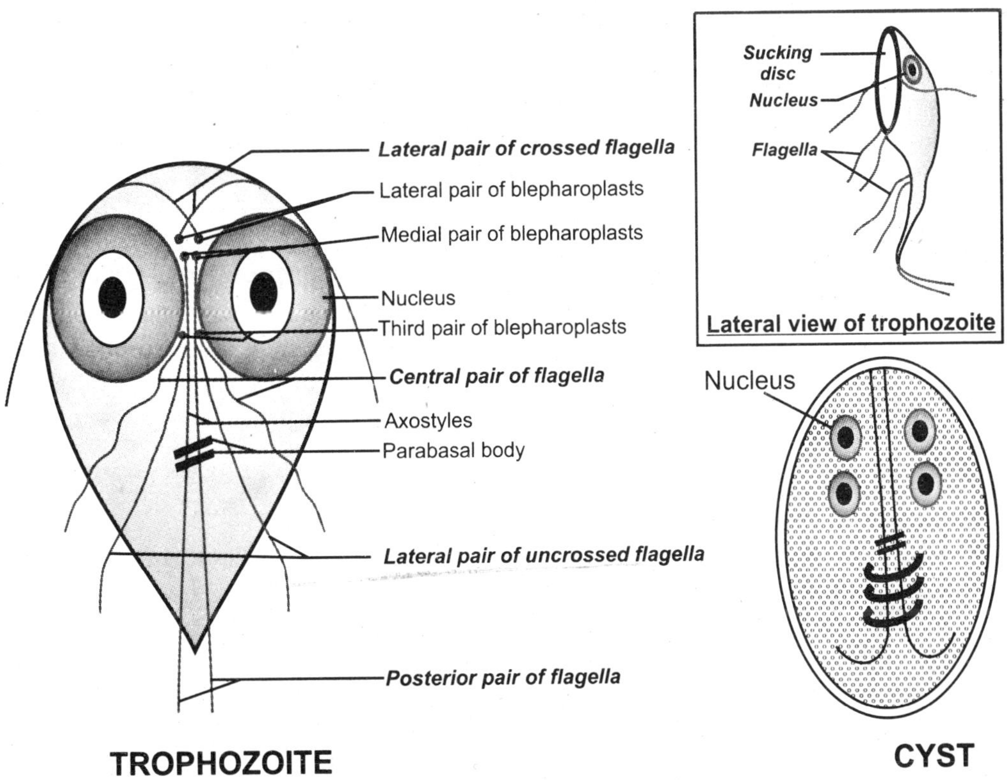

Fig. 22.3. Morphological forms of *Giarda lamblia.*

Cryptosporidium parvum

Oocyst is colourless, spherical or oval and measures 4–5 μm in diameter. It contains four crescent shaped naked or nonencysted sporozoites (sporocysts not present). The anterior end of the sporozoite is pointed and the posterior end which contains a prominent nucleus is rounded. The oocyst wall of *C. parvum* is composed of an electron-lucent middle zone surrounded by two electron-dense layers. Oocyst does not stain with iodine and is acid-fast (Colour Plate IV, Fig. 23).

Discussion

1. **Which morphlogical form of *E.histolytica* is seen in the tissues?**
   Trophozoite
2. **Define the term 'ameoboma.'**
   Amoeboma is pseudotumoural lesion caused by *E. histolytica* whose formation is associated with necrosis, inflammation and oedma of the mucosa and submucosa of the colon.
3. **What is the appearance of pus of liver abscess produced by *E. histolytica*?**
   Anchovy sauce
4. **What is the shape of trophozoite of *Giardia lamblia*?**
   Pear-shape
5. **How many pairs of blepharoplasts are present in trophozoite of *Giardia lamblia*?**
   Four
6. **What is the appearance of oocysts of *Cryptosporidium parvum* in modified acid-fast staining?**
   Red
7. **Enumerate parasites causing diarrhoeal disease in persons with HIV infection.**
   - *C. parvum*
   - *C. cayetanensis*
   - *I. belli*
   - Microsporidia
   - *E. histolytica*
   - *G. lamblia*
8. **Enumerate parasites causing traveller's diarrhoea.**
   - *E. histolytica*
   - *G. lamblia*
   - *C. cayetanensis*
   - *C. parvum*
9. **Enumerate parasites causing infection by ingestion of contaminated food and water.**
   - *E. histolytica*
   - *G. lamblia*
   - *C. cayetanensis*
   - *C. parvum*
   - *I. belli*
   - *B. coli*
10. **Enumerate protozoans causing CNS infection.**
    - *E. histolytica*
    - *Naegleria fowleri*
    - *Acanthamoeba* spp.
    - *Balamuthia mandrillaris*
    - Microsporidia
11. **Enumerate parasites causing dysentery.**
    - *E. histolytica*
    - *B. coli*
    - *Schistosoma japonicum*
    - *Trichuris trichiura*
12. **Which protozoan is associated with malabsorption syndrome?**
    G. lamblia
13. **Enumerate protozoans transmitted by sexual contact.**
    - *Trichomonas vaginalis*
    - *E. histolytica*
    - *G. lamblia*
14. **Which is the most common organ involved in extraintestinal amoebiasis?**
    Liver

Practical

23

Examination of Blood

The blood provides the most common medium for recovery of various stages of animal parasites e.g. *Plasmodium* spp., *Babesia* spp., *Leishmania* spp. *Trypanosoma brucei gambiense*, *Trypanosoma brucei rhodesiense*, *Trypanosoma cruzi, Wuchereria bancrofti* , *Brugia malayi, Brugia timori, Loa loa* and *Mansonella ozzardi*. However, in any particular infection the parasites may not be consistently present. Following methods can be used for the examination of parasites in the blood:

Wet preparation

A drop of anticoagulated blood can be placed on a clean glass slide, a cover-slip put in place and examined microscopically for large, often motile, exoerythrocytic parasites, such as trypanosomes and microfilariae.

Permanent stained blood smear

Permanent stained blood smear is essential for accurate identification of blood parasites. Two types of blood films are used:

- Thin blood film
- Thick blood film
- Combined thick and thin films on the same slide (Fig. 23.1)

Fig. 23.1. Combined thick and thin films on the same slide.

Thin blood film

Thin blood film is used primarily for the definitive species identification of plasmodia (Colour Plate V, Fig. 25) and other intraerythrocytic parasites. The pulp of a finger or lobe of an ear is wiped with spirit and allowed to dry. Thereafter, it is pricked with surgical cutting needle under aseptic condition. A drop of blood, about the size of pin head, is taken on a grease-free clean glass slide at about 2 cm from the right end. The drop of blood is touched with the edge of another slide. It is held at an angle of 30 degrees and pushed gently to the left, till the blood is exhausted. As the blood is exhausted, the film begins to form "tails" which end near about the centre of the slide. The film is allowed to dry. The thin film ideally is one cell thick, with erythrocytes lying flat on the glass surface. If the stain to be used is in an aqueous solution e.g. Giemsa stain, the film must be fixed by covering it with absolute methyl or ethyl alcohol for 2–3 minutes to prevent dehaemoglobinization. For alcohol stains e.g. Leishman stain, this treatment is not required.

Thick blood film

Thick blood film, many cells thick, contains 6–20 times as much blood per unit area as a thin film. A thick drop of blood is taken on a slide and spread with a needle or with a corner of another slide to form an area of about 12 mm square. It may also be prepared by taking four small drops of blood and joining the corners of the drop with a needle. The blood is continuously stirred for about 30 seconds to prevent formation of fibrin clots. If anticoagulated blood is used, stirring is not necessary because fibrin strands do not form. Potassium EDTA is the anticoagulant of choice. The film is allowed to air-dry in the dust-free area.The thickness of the film should be such as to allow a newsprint to be read or the hands of the wrist-watch to be seen through the dry preparation.

Once the film is dry, it should be dehaemoglobinized by placing the film in distilled water in a vertical position in a glass cylinder for 5–10 minutes. When the film becomes white, it is taken out and allowed to dry in an upright position. The disruption of the erythrocytes and the loss of their haemoglobin from the slide permits the remaining structures, including blood parasites, to be seen microscopically even when lying deep in the film. Dehaemoglobinization should be done as promptly as possible to assure total dehaemoglobinization. Thick blood films are especially useful in detecting malaria parasites in light infections.

Combined thick and thin films on the same slide

This method is of special value in survey work. Two drops of blood are taken; one, one cm and another, 2.5 cm from the right end of the slide. The former is made into a thick film and the latter into a thin film.

Staining blood film

Both thin and thick smears can be stained by Leishman and Giemsa stains. In addition, thick smear can be stained by Field Stain.

Discussion

1. **Enumerate the parasites which can be detected in peripheral blood smear.**
   - Malaria parasites
   - *Leishmania* spp.
   - Microfilariae
   - *Babesia* spp.
   - Trypanosomes
2. **Which organ is preferred for collection of blood in infants?**

   Big toe or heal is used for collection of blood in infants.
3. **Why blood should not be 'milked' out from the finger after finger is pricked?**

   This will dilute the blood with tissue fluids and hence will decrease the number of parasites per field.
4. **What is the advantage of preparation of thin blood film?**

   Thin blood film is used for the definitive species identification of plasmodia and other intraerythrocytic parasites.
5. **How do you identify a well prepared thin film?**
   - A well prepared thin film is thick at one end and thin at the other (one layer of evenly distributed RBCs with no cell overlap).
   - The thin, feathered end should be at least 2 cm long.
   - Thin film should occupy the central area of the slide, with free margins on both side.
6. **What problem can arise if you use a greasy slide?**

   Blood film spreads unevenly on a greasy slide.
7. **Why should heat fixation of blood film be avoided?**

   Because heat will fix the blood, causing the RBCs to remain intact during staining; the result is stain retention and inability to identify the parasites.
8. **What is the advantage of preparation of thick blood films?**

   Thick blood films are useful in detecting haemoparasites in light infection.
9. **What problem can arise if you use too much blood for preparing blood films?**

   In case of thin smear separate RBCs may not be available for examination and we may miss some parasites and in case of thick smear too many WBCs may interfere the diagnosis (obscure the parasites).
10. **What problem can arise if you use too little blood?**

    We may miss the infection.
11. **What is the advantage of combined thick and thin films on the same slide?**

    This method is useful in survey work.
12. **Which step is essential prior to staining of thick blood film?**

    Laking of thick smears is essential to remove haemoglobin before staining is done.
13. **What is the advantage of dehaemoglobinization of thick blood films?**

    Dehaemoglobinization permits the remaining structures, including blood parasites, to be seen microscopically even when lying deep in the film.

14. **Enumerate various stains for staining of blood films.**
    - Leishman
    - Giemsa
    - Field
    - J.S.B. (Jaswant Singh, Bhattacharjee) stain
15. **Why should you examine the feathered end of the blood film most carefully?**
    - Microfilariae are commonly found at the feathered end of the film, because they are carried to these sites during the process of spreading the blood.
    - Morphology and size of infected RBCs are most clearly seen as RBCs are drawn out into one single, distinctive layer of cells at this site.
    - Malaria parasites and trypanosomes are easily seen at the edges of thin film.
16. **At what time blood should be collected in cases of nocturnal filarial infections?**

    Blood should be collected during night, optimally between 10 p.m. and 2 a.m.
17. **Enumerate the microfilariae with sheaths.**
    - *Wuchereria bancrofti*
    - *Brugia malayi*
    - *Loa loa*
18. **In which microfilariae, tail-tip is free of nuclei?**
    - *W. bancrofti*
    - *Onchocerca volvulus*
    - *Mansonella ozzardi*
19. **Which blood film should be examined first if you are provided with thick and thin blood films?**

    Thin blood film should be examined first and if malaria parasite is seen then there is no need to examine thick film. But if you examine thick film first and you find malaria parasites then for species identification thin film is also examined.
20. **Which species of *Plasmodium* is most pathogenic?**

    P. falciparum
21. **Which species of *Plasmodium* are common in India?**

    P. vivax and P. falciparum
22. **In which malaria parasite infection only ring stage and gametocytes are seen in peripheral blood smear and why?**

    P. falciparum infection because other stages are sequestrated in the capillaries of internal organ.
23. **What is the shape of *P. falciparum* gametocytes?**

    Crescent shape
24. **Young RBCs are infected by which malaria parasites?**

    P. vivax and *P. ovale*
25. **The infected RBCs are enlarged due to infection by which malaria parasite?**

    P. vivax
26. **Relapse of malaria is seen due to infection by which parasite?**

    P. vivax and *P. ovale*
27. **What are the complications of *P. falciparum* infection?**

    Pernicious malaria and blackwater fever
28. **Which is the gold standard test for the detection of malaria parasites?**

    Peripheral blood smear examination

PART–4

Systemic Bacteriology

Contents

Practical 24

Staphylococcus

Introduction

Staphylococcus, *Micrococcus* and *Planococcus* belong to family Micrococcaceae. Genus *Staphylococcus* contains nearly 33 defined species, 20 of which are known to be associated with colonization and/or infection of man and animals. Of the 20 species, one (*Staphylococcus aureus)* is coagulase-positive and 19 are coagulase-negative.

Staphylococcus aureus

Morphology

They are Gram-positive, spherical cocci about 0.8–1.0 µm in diameter, arranged characteristically in grape-like clusters (Fig. 24.1). They are non-motile, non-sporing and with the exception of rare strains, non-capsulated.

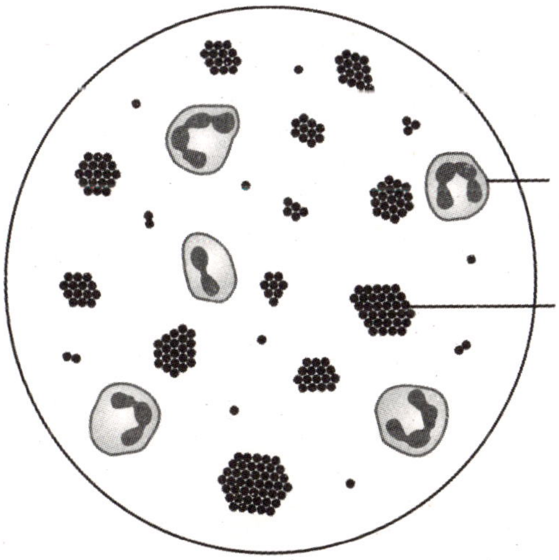

Fig. 24.1. Staphylococci in Gram-stained smear of pus.

Cultural characteristics

They are aerobes and facultative anaerobes. Optimum temperature for growth is 37°C, range being 12–44°C. Optimum pH is 7.5. They can grow well on ordinary media.

Nutrient agar

After overnight incubation at 37°C, colonies are 1–2 mm in diameter with a smooth glistening surface. They are opaque and easily emulsifiable. Most strains produce golden-yellow (aureus) pigment, though some strains may form white colonies.

Blood agar

Colonies are similar to those on nutrient agar, but may be surrounded by a zone of β-haemolysis (Colour Plate VI, Fig. 27), especially when the medium contains sheep, ox, or rabbit blood and it is incubated in an atmosphere of 20% CO_2. Haemolysis is weak on horse blood agar.

MacConkey agar

Colonies are smaller and pink due to lactose fermentation.

Mannitol salt agar

This is both selective and indicator medium. Colonies are similar to those on nutrient agar, but they are surrounded by yellow zones due to fermentation of mannitol by most strains of *S. aureus*.

Phenolphthalein phosphate agar

This is an indicator medium. This assists in the identification of *S. aureus* in mixed cultures. Colonies are similar to those on nutrient agar. All strains of *S. aureus* produce phosphatase which liberates phenolphthalein from sodium phenolphthalein diphosphate. To detect it, 0.1 ml of ammonia solution is placed in the lid and the culture plate, with the culture, is inverted over it. Colonies of *S. aureus* become bright pink in a minute or so because phenolphthalein is pink in alkaline pH.

Biochemical reactions

Catalase	+
Oxidase	–
Indole	–
MR	+
VP	+
Urease	+
Nitrate reduction	+
Acid from	
glucose	+
maltose	+
lactose	+
sucrose	+
mannitol	+

Tests to detect the production of coagulase are:

1) **Slide coagulase test** : This test detects clumping factor (bound coagulase) which is a cell wall component that causes the organisms to clump when mixed with plasma. This factor reacts directly with fibrinogen in plasma, causing rapid cell clumping. It can be detected by emulsifying a few colonies of bacteria in a drop of normal saline on a clean glass slide and mixing it with a drop of rabbit plasma. Prompt clumping of the organisms indicates the presence of clumping factor. Positive and negative controls are also set up.

2) **Tube coagulase test**: This test detects an extracellular enzyme called coagulase. It activates a coagulase-reacting factor (CRF) normally present in plasma, causing the plasma to clot by conversion of fibrinogen to fibrin. To perform this test, 0.1 ml of an overnight broth culture is mixed with 0.5 ml of a 1 in 10 dilution of human or rabbit plasma. The mixture is incubated in a water-bath at 37°C for three to six hours. If positive, the plasma clots and does not flow when the tube is inverted. If clot does not appear it is left overnight at room temperature and re-examined. On continued incubation, the clot may be lysed by fibrinolysin produced by some strains. Controls with plasma alone, known coagulase-positive and coagulase-negative cultures must be set up with each batch of tests.

Coagulase-negative staphylococci

Coagulase-negative staphylococci (CNS) form part of the normal flora of the skin but may cause opportunistic infection in immunocompromised patients. Their colonies are non-pigmented (white) (Colour Plate VI, Fig. 28), and in contrast to *S. aureus*, they are clumping factor, coagulase test and deoxyribonuclease negative. Majority (70–80%) of infections with CNS, in humans, are caused by *S. epidermidis* followed by *S. saprophyticus*, *S. haemolyticus*, *S. hominis* and *S. warneri*.

Discussion

1. **Name methods of enhancement of pigment production by *S. aureus*.**

   Pigment production is enhanced by following methods:
   - Addition of 1% glycerol monoacetate to nutrient agar
   - Using milk agar plate
   - Using fatty media such as Tween agar
   - Prolonged incubation
   - Leaving plates at room temperature

2. **Does pigment of *S. aureus* diffuse into the medium?**

   No

3. **What do you mean by term staphylococcus?**

   Staphyle in Greek meaning bunch of grapes and kokkos meaning a berry.

4. **Why salt agar is used as selective medium for isolation of staphylococci?**

   Salt agar is used as selective medium because staphylococci can grow in the presence of 10% or more of sodium chloride, while many other bacteria are inhibited at this concentration.

5. **Enumerate characteristic features of pathogenic strains of *S. aureus*.**

   Pathogenic strains of *S. aureus* usually exhibit the following features:
   - Coagulase-positive
   - Ferment mannitol
   - Produce golden-yellow pigment
   - Liquefy gelatin
   - Produce phosphatase
   - β-haemolysis on blood agar medium

6. **Why staphylococci are arranged characteristically in grape-like clusters?**
Cluster formation is due to cell division occurring in more than one plane with daughter cells remaining close together.

7. **What is protein A?**
Protein A is a cell wall component which binds to Fc region of IgG molecules leaving specific Fab sites free to combine with specific antigen. It is involved in coagglutination test.

8. **What do you mean by term clumping factor?**
Clumping factor (bound coagulase) is a surface component that causes the organisms to clump when mixed with plasma. This factor reacts directly with fibrinogen in plasma, causing rapid cell clumping. Here fibrinogen is not converted into fibrin.

9. **What is the principle of tube coagulase test?**
S. aureus produces an extracellular enzyme called coagulase. It activates a coagulase-reacting factor (CRF) normally present in plasma, causing plasma to clot by the conversion of fibrinogen to fibrin.

10. **Why guinea-pig plasma cannot be used for tube coagulase test?**
Plasma of guinea-pig lack CRF. So it cannot be used for detecting free coagulase.

11. **What is the role of coagulase in pathogenesis?**
Coagulase may act to coat the bacterial cells with fibrin, rendering them resistant to opsonization and phagocytosis.

12. **Why citrated plasma should not be used for conducting tube coagulase test?**
Citrated plasma should not be used because contaminating Gram-negative bacilli may utilize the citrate and produce false positive reaction.

13. **Enumerate the pathogenic lesions produced by *S. aureus*.**
    - *Cutaneous infections* : Boils, furuncles, carbuncles, styes, etc.
    - *Deep infections* : Osteomyelitis ,tonsillitis ,bronchopneumonia, meningitis, etc.
    - *Exfoliative diseases* : Ritter's disease and staphylococcal scalded skin syndrome
    - Food poisoning
    - Toxic shock syndrome

14. **Which toxins of *S. aureus* are recognized as superantigens?**
    - Toxic shock syndrome toxin-1 (TSST-1)
    - Enterotoxins

15. **How much time after consuming contaminated food, patient develops staphylococcal food poisoning ?**
Within 2–6 hours

16. **What are the characteristic features of enterotoxins produced by *S. aureus*?**
    - Heat-stable
    - Not destroyed by gut enzymes
    - They act directly on autonomic nervous system to cause the illness, rather than on gastrointestinal mucosa.

17. **Why human blood should not be used for preparation of blood agar plate?**
Human blood should not be used because of following reasons:
    - Human blood may contain antibodies or other inhibitors.
    - α-lysin produced by *S. aureus* does not lyse human red blood cells.
    - Activity of β-lysin is weak on human red blood cells.

18. **Which haemolysin is known as hot-cold haemolysin?**
β-lysin

19. **Which species of coagulase-negative staphylococci is associated with urinary tract infection in young healthy sexually active women?**
S. saprophyticus

20. **Name one important test to differentiate *S. saprophyticus* from *S. aureus* and *S. epidermidis*.**
Novobiocin resistance test. *S. saprophyticus* is resistant to novobiocin while *S. aureus* and *S. epidermidis* are sensitive.

21. **Differentiate between *S. aureus* and *S. epidermidis*.**

	S. aureus	*S. epidermidis*
Production of		
Coagulase	+	–
DNase	+	–
α toxin	+	–
Phosphatase	+	–/weak +
Protein A in cell wall	+	–
Mannitol fermentation	+	–

22. **Enumerate organisms producing black colonies on blood tellurite agar medium.**
    - *Corynebacterium diphtheriae*
    - *S. aureus*
    - Enterococci

23. **What is the mechanism of resistance to β-lactam drugs in *S. aureus*?**
    - Production of β-lactamase
    - Changes in bacterial surface receptors reducing binding of β-lactam antibiotics to the bacterial cells
    - Development of tolerance

24. **Differentiate between bound coagulase and free coagulase of *S. aureus*.**

Bound coagulase	*Free coagulase*
• Cell wall component	• Extracellular enzyme
• Only one antigen type is known	• Eight antigenic types have been identified
• Does not require participation of coagulase-reacting factor	• Requires the participation of coagulase-reacting factor for its action
• Detected by slide coagulase test	• Detected by tube coagulase test

Practical 25

Streptococcus pyogenes, S. agalactiae and Enterococci

Introduction

On the basis of group-specific carbohydrate antigen in the cell wall, β-haemolytic streptococci are divided into 21 serological groups. These are known as Lancefield groups. Group A β-haemolytic strains, which are responsible for many important human infections, are given the species name *Streptococcus pyogenes*.

Streptococcus pyogenes

Morphology

They are Gram-positive, spherical cocci about 0.6–1.0 μm in diameter. They occur in chains of varying length (Fig. 25.1). They are non-motile, non-sporing and some strains produce a capsule of hyaluronic acid.

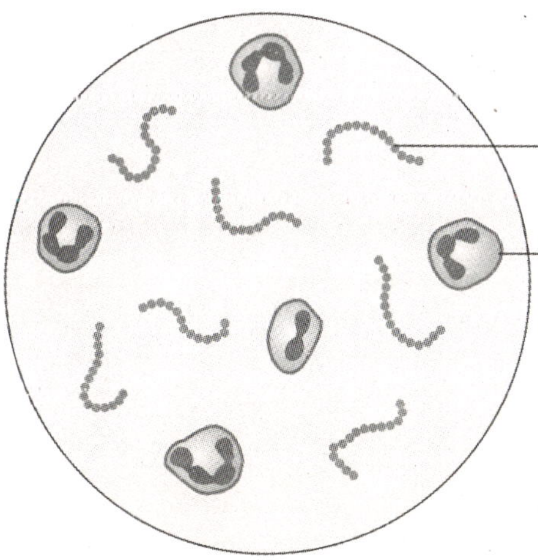

Fig. 25.1. Streptococci in Gram-stained smear of pus.

Cultural characteristics

They are aerobes and facultative anaerobes. Temperature range is 22–40°C, optimum temperature being 37°C. They are exacting in nutritive requirements, growth occurring only in media containing fermentable carbohydrates or enriched with blood or serum.

Blood agar

After 24 hours incubation, colonies are small (0.5–1 mm), semitransparent, grey-white with a matt or glossy surface. The colonies are surrounded by a wide zone of β-haemolysis (Colour Plate VI, Fig. 29). Mucoid colonies are formed by strains which produce large capsule. On ageing and drying, mucoid colonies turn into flatter, rougher, matt colonies. Growth and haemolysis are promoted by 10% CO_2.

Crystal violet blood agar

This is a selective medium for isolation of *S. pyogenes*. The addition of 0.0002% crystal violet to blood agar inhibits the growth of some bacteria, notably staphylococci, while permitting the growth of streptococci.

PNF medium

This is a selective medium for β-haemolytic streptococci. It inhibits the growth of staphylococci and coliform species.

Glucose broth or serum broth

These are liquid media used for isolation of streptococci. Growth occurs as granular turbidity with a powdery deposit. No pellicle is formed.

Biochemical reactions

Catalase	–
Solubility in 10% bile	–
Sensitivity to	
bacitracin disc (0.04 μg)	+
trimethoprim/sulphamethoxazole (1.2 μg/23.8 μg)	–

Group B streptococci (Streptococcus agalactiae)

Morphology

They are chain forming Gram-positive cocci. They are non-motile and non-sporing.

Cultural characteristics

Blood agar

On blood agar, they produce β-haemolysis, though the zones are usually narrow. Sometime they may produce α-haemolysis and occasionally they produce no haemolysis at all. Colonies are grey, mucoid and larger (about 2 mm) than those of other streptococci.

Columbia agar or starch/serum agar

They form orange-coloured colonies on anaerobic incubation at 37°C for 18 hours.

Islam medium

Pigment production is more intense on this medium.

Tests for presumptive identification of group B streptococci

Hydrolysis of sodium hippurate

S. agalactiae possesses the enzyme hippuricase, which hydrolyzes sodium hippurate to form sodium benzoate and glycine. This hydrolysis can be detected by adding ninhydrin, which reacts with the α-amino groups to form a purple colour. All group B streptococci hydrolyze hippurate.

CAMP test

This test detects the production of CAMP factor produced by group B streptococci. CAMP factor enhances the β-lysin produced by *Staphylococcus*.

To perform this test, streak a β-lysin-producing *Staphylococcus aureus* strain (NCTC 1803) on a sheep blood agar plate. Then make a single streak of the streptococcal test strain perpendicular to the staphylococcal streak. Leave about 1 cm space between the two inoculation lines. Incubate the inoculated plate at 37°C for 24 hours in air or in air with 10% CO_2. CAMP factor enhances the β-lysin produced by *Staphylococcus* and an increased area of lysis appears at the junction of the two organisms which assume the shape of an arrowhead (Fig. 25.2).

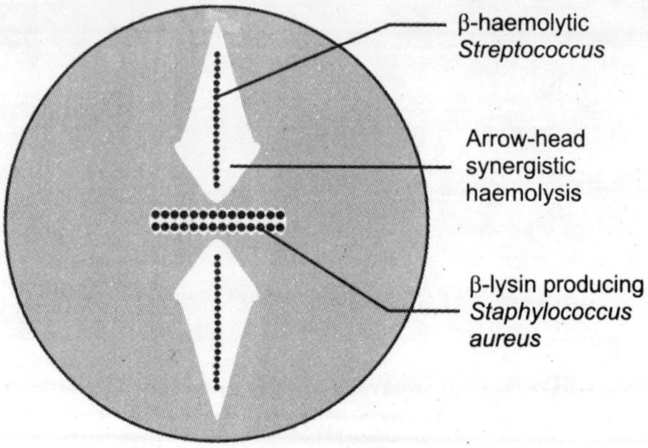

Fig. 25.2. CAMP test.

Enterococcus

They are Gram-positive cocci occurring in pairs or short chains. They are non-motile and non-capsulated. They are normal flora of lower GIT and vagina. They may be α, β or non-haemolytic on sheep blood agar. They produce tiny, deep pink colonies on MacConkey agar.

Important characteristics of enterococci are :

- They can grow in the presence of 40% bile and hydrolyze aesculin to aesculetin and glucose.
- They can grow in the presence of 6.5% NaCl, at pH 9.6, and at 10°C and 45°C.
- They are positive for PYRase test.
- They can tolerate heat at 60°C for 30 minutes.
- They are resistant to penicillin.

Discussion

1. **What is the basis of Lancefield classification of β-haemolytic streptococci?**
   Lancefield classification is based on the nature of group-specific carbohydrate antigens in the cell wall.
2. **What do you mean by Griffith typing of group A streptococci?**
   Group A streptococci may be further subdivided into types based on protein (M,T and R) antigens present on the cell surface. More than 120 M types of *S. pyogenes* have been recognized so far (types 1,2,3 and so on). This is known as Griffith typing.

3. **Why there is chain formation in streptococci?**
   Chain formation is due to the cocci dividing in one plane only and the daughter cells failing to separate completely.

4. **Name one longest chain forming *Streptococcus*.**
   S. salivarius

5. **How many types of haemolysis are seen in streptococci?**
   Three types of haemolysis are seen :
   - Alpha
   - Beta
   - Gamma

6. **Enumerate non-suppurative complications of *S. pyogenes*.**
   - Acute rheumatic fever
   - Acute glomerulonephritis
   - Erythema nodosum

7. **Name one transport medium used for isolation of streptococci.**
   Pike's medium (blood agar containing 1 in 1,000,000 crystal violet and 1 in 16,000 sodium azide distributed as for stab cultures in tubes).

8. **Enumerate pathogenic lesions produced by group B streptococci.**
   In neonates
   - Early-onset-type meningitis
   - Late-onset-type meningitis

   In adults
   - Puerperal sepsis
   - Endocarditis
   - Meningitis
   - Occasionally pneumonia, empyema, arthritis and osteomyelitis

9. **Name presumptive tests for identification of group B streptococci.**
   - Hydrolysis of sodium hippurate
   - CAMP test
   - Pigment production

10. **Who first described the CAMP test?**
    CAMP test was first described in 1944 by Christie, Atkins and Munch-Peterson.

11. **Name streptococci responsible for dental caries.**
    Viridans streptococci, chiefly *S. mutans* and to a lesser extent *S. sanguis*, are involved in the production of dental caries.

12. **Describe in brief the mechanism of dental caries.**
    Viridans streptococci, chiefly *S. mutans* and to a lesser extent *S. sanguis* break down dietary sucrose, producing acid and a tough adhesive dextran. The acid damages dentine and the dextran bind together food debris, epithelial cells, mucus and bacteria to form dental plaques which lead to dental caries.

13. **Enumerate viridans streptococci associated with infective endocarditis.**
    - *S. mutans*
    - *S. sanguis*
    - *S. salivarius*
    - *S. mitior*
    - *S. milleri*

14. **What is the typical arrangement of enterococci?**
    Enterococci typically appear as pairs of oval cocci, the cells in a pair are arranged at an angle to each other.

15. **What is the therapeutic role of streptokinase and streptodornase (deoxyribonuclease) produced by streptococci?**
    Mixtures of streptokinase and streptodornase have been used therapeutically for breaking down blood clots, thick pus and fibrinous exudates in closed spaces such as joints or pleural cavity.

16. **Which enzymes of group A streptococci are responsible for serous character of pus?**
    Deoxyribonucleases

17. **Enumerate structural components of *S. pyogenes* which cross-react with human tissues.**

Structural component of *S. pyogenes*	Human tissue with which it cross-reacts
Capsular hyaluronic acid	Synovial fluid
Cell wall protein	Myocardium
Cell wall carbohydrate	Cardiac valves
Cytoplasmic membrane	Vascular intima
Peptidoglycan	Skin antigens

18. **Which test can differentiate streptococci from staphylococci?**
    Catalase test, the former are negative and the latter are positive.

19. **Which *Streptococcus* is strict anaerobe?**
    Peptostreptococcus

20. **What is the major difference between lesions produced by staphylococci and streptococci?**
    Staphylococci produce localized lesions while streptococci produce spreading lesions.

Practical 26

Streptococcus Pneumoniae (Pneumococcus)

Morphology

Pneumococci are small (1 μm), slightly elongated Gram-positive cocci, with one end broad or rounded and the other pointed, presenting a flame-shaped or lanceolate appearance. They occur in pairs with rounded ends adjacent to each other. They are capsulated. The capsule encloses each pair and it is best seen in the material taken directly from the exudates and may be lost on repeated cultivation (Fig. 26.1). They are non-motile and non-sporing.

Cultural characteristics

They are aerobes and facultative anaerobes, the optimum temperature being 37°C (range 25–40°C) and pH 7.8 (range 6.5–8.3). They grow only in enriched media and growth is improved by 5–10% CO_2.

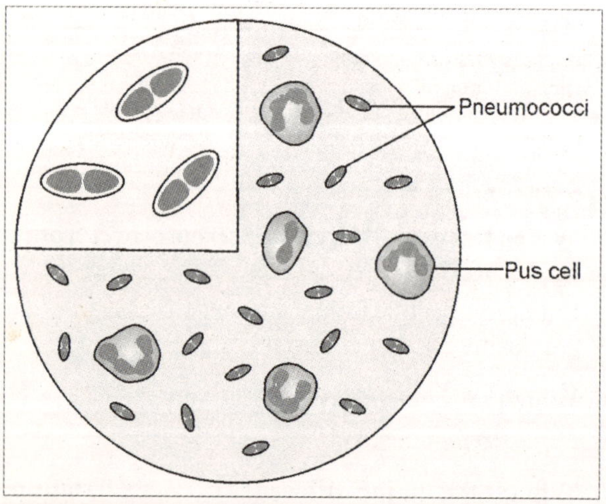

Fig. 26.1. Pneumococci in pus inset : enlarged view.

Blood agar

Virulent strains with abundant capsular polysaccharide produce small (0.5–1 mm in diameter), moist, mucoid, transparent colonies after 18–24 hours incubation at 37°C. Poorly capsulated strains produce small, round, translucent colonies. The colonies are surrounded by a 2–3 mm zone of α-haemolysis (Colour Plate VI, Fig. 30). On further incubation, the colonies develop a central depression because of autolysis with raised rim (draughtsman çolony). Under anaerobic incubation, β-haemolysis is seen due to the liberation of oxygen-labile pneumolysin by pneumococci.

Biochemical rections

Catalase	–
Acid from	
glucose	+
sucrose	+
lactose	+
inulin	+
Bile solubility	+

Fermentation reactions are tested in Hiss's serum water.

Tests for indentification of pneumococci

1) Optochin sensitivity

Optochin (ethyl hydrocuprein hydrochloride) is a quinine derivative that inhibits the growth of pneumococci. For testing, a filter paper disc (5μg) of optochin is applied to the surface of a blood agar plate streaked with a lawn of pure culture. Plate is incubated at 37°C in air with 5–10% CO_2. Pneumococcus shows a zone of inhibition of 14 mm or more around the 6 mm optochin disc or 16 mm or more if 10 mm disc is used. This test is also used for distinguishing pneumococci from viridans streptococci, both of which produce α-haemolysis on blood agar. Viridans streptococci are resistant to optochin.

2) Bile solubility

For bile solubility test, inoculate the test organism in 5 ml serum digest broth or infusion broth, incubate it at 37°C for 18 hours. While still warm, add 0.5 ml of 10% sodium deoxycholate solution and reincubate at 37°C. Within 15 minutes initially turbid culture becomes clear and transparent due to the lysis of pneumococci. Alternatively, touch a suspected pneumococcal colony on blood agar plate with a loopful of 2% sodium deoxycholate solution at pH 7. Incubate the plate at 37°C for 30 minutes. The colony disappears, leaving an area of α-haemolysis.

Discussion

1) **Enumerate methods for the demonstration of capsule of pneumoccoci.**
   - A clear halo around the organism in India ink preparation
   - By direct special staining techniques
   - It can also be seen and typed by treatment with homologous type-specific antibody which combines with the capsular polysaccharide and renders it refractile – Quellung reaction.

2) **What is the historical importance of pneumococci?**
   Research work with pneumococcal transformations provided the initial proof that DNA alone is the carrier of genetic information.

3) **Which type of haemolysis is seen in pneumococci?**
   α-haemolysis

4) **How do you differentiate *S. pneumoniae* from viridans streptococci?**

	S. pneumoniae	Viridans streptococci
• Morphology	Flame-shaped cocci in pairs	oval or round cocci in chains
• Capsule	Present	Absent
• Bile solubility	+	–
• Inulin fermentation	+	–
• Optochin sensitivity	+	–
• Animal pathogenicity (intraperitoneal inoculation in mice)	Fatal, death of mice in 1–3 days	Nonpathogenic

5) **What name is given to the colonies of *S. pneumoniae*?**
   Draughtman colonies or colonies with carrom coin appearance. The colonies are flat with raised edges and central umbonation.

6) **Enumerate pathogenic lesions produced by *S. pneumoniae.***
   - Pneumonia, either a lobarpneumonia or a bronchopneumonia
   - Bronchitis
   - Sinusitis
   - Otitis media
   - Meningitis
   - Endocarditis
   - Suppurative arthritis
   - Peritonitis

7) **Name the commonest pneumococcal infections.**
   Otitis media and sinusitis.

Practical 27

Neisseria

Introduction

The genus *Neisseria* has Gram-negative cocci with adjacent sides flattened. They are saccharolytic, catalase-positive and oxidase-positive. *N. gonorrhoeae* and *N. meningitidis* are the primary human pathogens of the genus. Other species are commonly found as commensals in the upper respiratory tract.

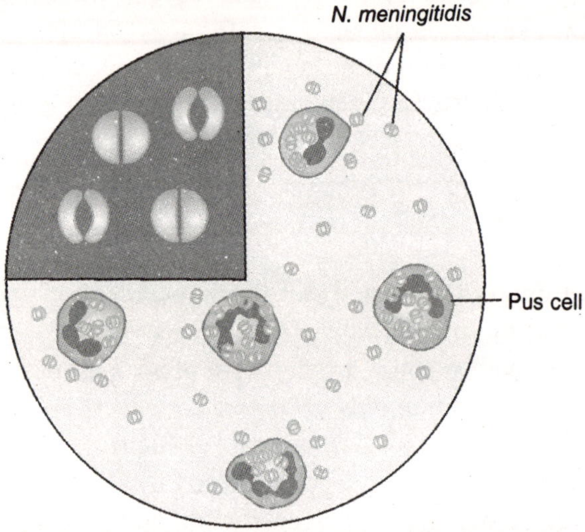

Fig. 27.1. *Neisseria meningitidis* in CSF. Inset : enlarged view showing adjacent sides flattened or concave and long axes parallel.

Neisseria meningitidis (meningococcus)

Morphology

They are Gram-negative cocci, 0.6–1.0 µm in diameter. They usually occur in pairs with adjacent sides flattened or concave and long axes parallel. They are typically seen in large numbers inside polymorphonuclear leucocytes (Fig. 27.1). Fresh isolates of most *N. meningitidis* serogroups are encapsulated. They are non-sporing and non-motile.

Cultural characteristics

Meningococci have exacting growth requirements and do not grow on ordinary media. Growth occurs on media enriched with blood or serum. However, they grow well on trypticase-soy agar and Mueller-Hinton medium without the addition of blood or serum. They are strict aerobes, no growth occurring anaerobically. The growth is facilitated by 5–10% CO_2 and high humidity. The optimum temperature and pH for the growth of meningococci are 35–36°C and 7.0–7.4 respectively.

Blood agar

On blood agar, after 24 hours incubation, the colonies of meningococci are small about 1 mm in diameter, round, convex, grey, non-haemolytic and translucent. After 48 hours incubation, colonies are larger with an opaque raised centre and thin transparent margins which may be crenated.

Chocolate agar

Colonies of meningococci are slightly larger than those on blood agar.

Thayer-Martin medium

This is a selective medium for the growth of gonococci and meningococci. This medium is used for the culture of materials expected to yield a mixture of organisms. Vancomycin, colistin and nystatin which are present in this medium inhibit Gram-positive bacteria, Gram-negative bacteria and yeast contaminants respectively, while allowing the growth of pathogenic *Neisseria*.

Biochemical Reactions

Catalase	+
Oxidase	+
Acid from	
glucose	+
maltose	+

Neisseria gonorrhoeae (gonococcus)

Morphology and staining characteristics of *N. gonorrhoeae* are similar to those of *N. meningitidis*.

Cultural characteristics

Gonococci are more difficult to grow than meningococci. They are aerobes, but may grow anaerobically. Addition of 5–10% CO_2 is essential for primary isolation. Growth occurs best at pH 7.0–7.4 and at a temperature of 35–36°C. They can be isolated on media enriched with blood, either partially lysed by heat (chocolate agar) or completely lysed by saponin.

Heated blood agar

On heated blood agar, after 24 hours incubation, colonies are small about 1 mm in diameter, grey, convex and translucent. After 48 hours incubation, colonies are larger 1.5–2.5 mm in diameter with an opaque raised centre and thin transparent margins which may be crenated.

Thayer-Martin medium

This is a selective medium for gonococci. This is prepared by addition of vancomycin 3 mg/litre, colistin 7.5 mg/litre and nystatin 12,500 units/litre to heated blood agar. This selective medium is valuable in isolating gonococci from heavily contaminated specimens. On Thayer-Martin medium growth is slower, although colonies are similar to those on heated blood agar (Colour Plate VI, Fig. 31).

Modified Thayer-Martin medium

Trimethoprim lactate (5 mg/litre) may be added to Thayer-Martin medium to inhibit swarming *Proteus* species that are occasionally present in cervicovaginal and rectal specimens. The chocolate agar medium containing vancomycin, colistin, nystatin and trimethoprim is known as modified Thayer-Martin medium.

Biochemical reactions

Catalase	+
Oxidase	+
Acid from	
glucose	+
maltose	–

Discussion

1. **Enumerate important bacteria causing meningitis.**
   - Meningococci
   - Pneumococci
   - *Haemophilus influenzae* type b
   - Group B streptococci
   - *Listeria monocytogenes*
2. **Name one transport medium for *Neisseria meningitidis*.**

   Stuart's medium
3. **Which site acts as a reservoir of meningococci?**

   The human nasopharynx is the only reservoir of meningococci.
4. **Name oxidase-positive organisms.**
   - *Neisseria* spp.
   - *Alcaligenes faecalis*
   - *Aeromonas* spp.
   - *Vibrio* spp.
   - *Campylobacter* spp.
   - *Pseudomonas* spp.
5. **Which organ is the primary site of gonococcal infection in women?**

   In women, endocervix is the primary site of infection.
6. **Enumerate organisms causing non-gonococcal urethritis (NGU).**
   - *Chlamydia trachomatis*
   - *Ureaplasma urealyticum*
   - *Candida albicans*
   - *Mycoplasma genitalium*
   - *Gardnerella vaginalis*
   - *Mycoplasma hominis*
   - *Trichomonas vaginalis*
7. **Enumerate pathogenic lesions caused by *N. meningitidis*.**
   - Meningitis
   - Septicaemia or meningococcaemia
   - Waterhouse-Friderichsen syndrome

Practical

28

Corynebacterium

Coryneform bacteria are pleomorphic, club-shaped, Gram-positive bacilli arranged in V forms or palisades. On the basis of cell wall composition and G+C content of DNA, the coryneform bacteria have been divided into 10 genera. The major pathogen in the genus *Corynebacterium* is *C. diphtheriae.*

Corynebacterium diphtheriae

Morphology

They are thin, slender, non-sporing, non-capsulated, non-motile, non-acid-fast, Gram-positive bacilli of varying lengths with an average size of 3×0.3 µm. They frequently possess club-shaped swellings at one or both ends, a characteristic feature which is responsible for the name of the genus (coryne means club). When dividing, the bacilli snap and bend abruptly and appear as angled pairs or parallel rows of 3–4 bacilli (palisades) which resemble Chinese letters (Fig. 28.1).

Although Gram-positive, *C. diphtheriae* is readily decolourized. Another characteristic of this organism is its granular and uneven staining. When stained with methylene blue or toluidine blue, the granules in the cell stain metachromatically reddish-purple. Most cells contain 2 or 3 of these, and they tend to be on the poles. With Albert stain, the granules stain bluish-black and the cytoplasm green.

Cultural characteristics

They are aerobes and facultative anaerobes. Optimum temperature for growth is 37°C (range 15–40°C). They can grow on ordinary nutrient agar, but their growth is improved by the presence of animal proteins such as serum or blood (Colour Plate VI, Fig. 32).

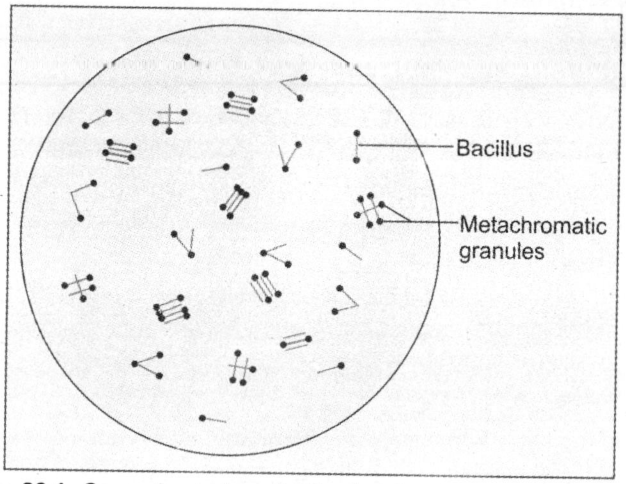

Fig. 28.1. *Corynebacterium diphtheriae* showing metachromatic granules and Chinese letter arrangement.

Loeffler's serum slope

Diphtheria bacilli grow rapidly on Loeffler's serum slope and colonies can be seen in 6–8 hours, long before other bacteria grow. The colonies are at first small, white, opaque discs, but on continued incubation increase in size and may acquire a yellow tint.

Blood tellurite agar (BTA)

The addition of 0.03–0.04% potassium tellurite to blood agar makes the medium selective for corynebacteria by inhibiting most other pathogenic and commensal bacteria. On this medium, colonies of *C. diphtheriae* become grey to black (Colour Plate VI, Fig. 33) because tellurite or tellurous ions are able to diffuse through the cell wall and membrane and are reduced to tellurium metal, which is precipitated inside the cell. On the basis of colonial morphology on BTA, diphtheria bacilli can be divided into three biotypes – mitis, intermedius and gravis.

Mitis : Colonies are grey, opaque, 1.5–2.0 mm in diameter with regular margins and glossy smooth surface. On further incubation the colony become flat with central elevation and regular margins – **'poached egg'** colony.

Intermedius : Small (0.5–0.75 mm in diameter), grey colony with darker centre and a shining surface – **'frog's egg'** colony. There is little change in size after 48 hours incubation.

Gravis : Colonies are dull greyish-black, opaque, 1.5–2.5 mm in dameter. In 2–3 days, 3–5 mm in diameter flat colony with raised dark centre, radially striated periphery and crenated edge – **'daisy-head'** colony.

Biochemical reactions

Catalase	+
Acid from	
glucose	+
maltose	+
H_2S production	+
Nitrate reduction	+

The fermentation tests are usually done by culture for 24 hours at 37°C in Hiss's serum peptone water medium.

Virulence tests of C. diphtheriae

These are of two types:

1. *In vitro.*
   - Elek's gel precipitation test
2. *In vivo (in guinea-pig or rabbit)*
   - Subcutaneous
   - Intradermal

Elek's gel precipitation test

This is a gel precipitation test. Pipette 10 ml of nutrient agar that has been cooled to 55°C in a water-bath and 2 ml sterile calf serum in a petri dish and rotate 20 times to mix. Before the medium solidifies, place a 1 cm × 8 cm filter paper strip that has been soaked in the diphtheria antitoxin 500–1,000 units/ml across the middle of the plate on the surface of the agar. Allow the medium to solidify and then place the plate in the incubator with the lid ajar to allow the surface moisture to evaporate. Inoculate the plate within 2 hours after drying by streaking a heavy inoculum of the culture to be tested across the plate at right angles to the antitoxin strip. Parallel to this streak, at a distance of about 15 mm from it, streak a known toxigenic strain of *C. diphtheriae* on one side of the test strain and streak a non-toxigenic strain on the other side.

Incubate the plate at 37°C and examine after 24 and 48 hours. Look for white lines of precipitation a few mm from the paper strip, that extend out from the line of bacterial growth, forming an angle of about 45°. These white precipitin lines form where the toxin from pathogenic strains of *C. diphtheriae* combines with antitoxin in an optimum concentration from the paper strip, thus identifying the strains of *C. diphtheriae* that produce toxin. Look for continuity between the lines from unknown culture and that from the known toxigenic culture (Fig. 28.2).

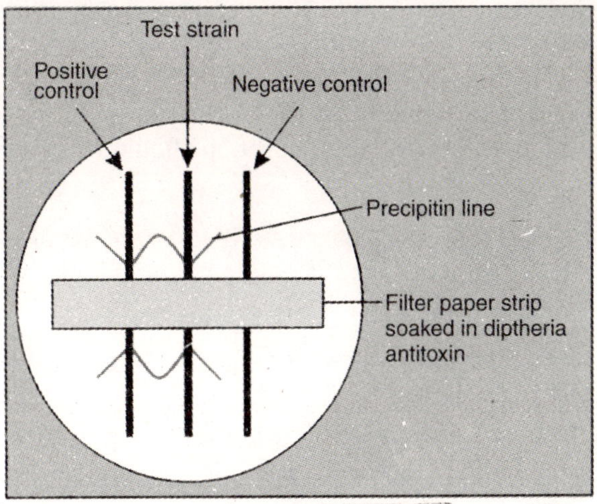

Fig. 28.2. Elek's test.

Discussion

1. **Which medium is used to obtain early growth of *C. diphtheriae*?**
   Loeffler's serum slope (LSS)
2. **Enumerate various advantages of Loeffler's serum slope.**
   - Growth of *C. diphtheriae* on LSS is obtained within 6–8 hours.
   - It is used for rich production of metachromatic granules.
   - It is used for growth of pure culture of *C. diphtheriae* for conducting toxigenicity test of *C. diphtheriae.*
3. **Name one selective medium for *C. diphtheriae.***
   Blood tellurite agar (BTA)
4. **Why does *C. diphtheriae* produce grey-black colonies on BTA?**
   On this medium, colonies of *C. diphtheriae* become grey to black because tellurite or tellurous ions are able to diffuse through the cell wall and membrane and are reduced to tellurium metal, which is precipitated inside the cell.

5. **Why *C. diphtheriae* colonies take 24–48 hours to grow on BTA medium?**
Potassium tellurite may retard the growth even of corynebacteria so that colonies may be very small after 24 hours, therefore, incubation should be continued for 48 hours.

6. **How many biotypes of *C. diphtheriae* are there?**
Three biotypes – mitis, intermedius and gravis

7. **Which biotype of *C. diphtheriae* ferments starch and glycogen?**
Gravis.

8. **Which biotype of *C. diphtheriae* produces β–haemolysis on sheep or rabbit blood agar plate?**
Mitis

9. **Why does *C. diphtheriae* show Chinese letter arrangement?**
When dividing, diphtheria bacilli snap and bend abruptly and appear as angled pairs or parallel rows of 3–4 bacilli which resemble Chinese letters. This arrangement is due to the incomplete separation of daughter cells after binary fission.

10. **What is the characteristic name given to the colony of 'mitis' biotype on BTA?**
'Poached egg' colony

11. **What is the mechanism of the necrotic and neurotoxic effects of diphtheria toxin?**
Inhibition of protein synthesis

12. **What are the constituents of pseudomembrane produced by *C. diphtheriae*?**
Necrotic cellular material, erythrocytes, fibrin, epithelial cells, leucocytes and bacteria

13. **Enumerate complications of diphtheria.**
    - Asphyxia due to mechanical obstruction of the respiratory passage by the pseudomembrane
    - Acute circulatory failure
    - Postdiphtheritic paralysis

14. **Name the sources of infection of *C. diphtheriae*.**
Carriers and symptomatic patients are the sources of infection. But carriers are more important than symptomatic patients.

15. **Name tissues for which diphtheria toxin has special affinity.**
    - Heart muscles
    - Nerve endings
    - Adrenal glands

16. **What is the immunization schedule of DPT?**
DPT (diphtheria toxoid in combination with tetanus toxoid and killed suspension of pertussis bacilli) is given at the age of 6 weeks, 10 weeks, 14 weeks and 16–24 months followed by DT at the age of 5–6 years.

17. **What is the advantage of combined preparation of DPT (triple vaccine)?**
    - It minimizes the number of injections.
    - It also improves immune response because the pertussis vaccine acts as an adjuvant for the toxoids.

18. **What is the role of antimicrobial agents in treatment of diphtheria?**
Antimicrobial agents kill diphtheria bacilli and prevent further toxin production.

Practical 29

Mycobacterium Tuberculosis

Morphology

Tubercle bacilli are slender, straight or slightly curved rods with rounded ends. They measure 1–4 × 0.2–0.8 µm (average 3 × 0.3 µm) in size. In sputum and other clinical specimens they may occur singly or in small clumps. True branching is occasionally seen in old cultures and in smears from caseous lymph nodes. They are non-motile, non-sporing, non-capsulated and acid-fast. The Ziehl-Neelsen acid-fast stain is useful in staining organisms from cultures or from clinical material. With this stain, the tubercle bacilli stain bright red, while the tissue cells and other organisms are stained blue (Colour Plate I, Fig. 3). Organisms in tissue and sputum smears often stain irregularly and have a beaded or barred appearance, presumably because of their vacuoles and polyphosphate content. Tubercle bacilli are Gram-positive but it is difficult to stain them with the Gram stain. This is because of the failure of the dye to penetrate the cell wall.

Cultural characteristics

Mycobacterium tuberculosis is an obligate aerobe. Optimum temperature for growth is 37°C and optimum pH is 7.0. Tubercle bacilli can grow on a wide range of enriched culture media but Lowenstein- Jensen (LJ) medium is most widely used. This medium consists of whole egg, asparagine, some mineral salts, malachite green and glycerol or sodium pyruvate and solidified by heating (inspissation). Lowenstein-Jensen glycerol medium is recommended for the isolation of human tubercle bacillus whose growth is enhanced by 0.75% glycerol but glycerol at this concentration is inhibitory to *M. bovis*, therefore, it may fail to grow on this medium. However, when the concentration of glycerol is reduced to 0.5% it still improves the growth of *M. tuberculosis* but generally does not inhibit the growth of *M. bovis*. Sodium pyruvate improves the growth of both *M. tuberculosis* and *M. bovis*. LJ medium may be made selective by addition of cycloheximide (400 µg/ml), lincomycin (2 µg/ml) and nalidixic acid (35 µg/ml) in addition to malachite green (0.025 g/ml), to suppress bacterial and fungal contaminants.

LJ medium

M. tuberculosis grows well on LJ medium (eugonic growth). It produces visible growth on LJ glycerol medium, incubated at 37°C, in about 2 weeks, although on primary isolation from clinical material, colonies may take up to 8 weeks to appear. It grows as rough, tough and buff colonies – rough due to dry, irregular growth, tough due to difficulty in lifting the colony from the surface, and buff due to the pale yellow colour (Colour Plate VI, Fig. 34).

Glycerol broth

In glycerol broth, the hydrophobic properties of the organisms cell surface result in a whitish wrinkled pellicle and granular deposit.

Biochemical reactions

1. Niacin accumulation

M. tuberculosis accumulates niacin as a water-soluble by-product in the culture medium.

2. Neutral red test

This test detects the ability of a strain to bind neutral red in an alkaline buffer solution. Positive tests are obtained with *M. tuberculosis, M. bovis* and *M. ulcerans.*

3. Catalase activity

M. tuberculosis is weakly catalase-positive.

4. Susceptibility to pyrazinamide

M. tuberculosis is sensitive to 50 µg/ml pyrazinamide.

5. Amidase test

M. tuberculosis produces nicotinamidase and pyrazinamidase.

6. Nitrate reduction test

M. tuberculosis produces enzyme nitroreductase. Therefore, it reduces nitrate to nitrite.

Discussion

1. **Who first isolated the mammalian tubercle bacilli and proved its causative role in tuberculosis?**
   Robert Koch (1882)
2. **Name organisms causing tuberculosis in humans.**
   - *M. tuberculosis*
   - *M. bovis*
   - *M. africanum*
3. **Name saprophytic mycobacteria.**
   - *M. butyricum*
   - *M. phlei*
   - *M. stercoris*
   - *M. smegmatis*
4. **Why does *M. tuberculosis* often stain irregularly and have beaded or barred appearance?**
   This is due to their vacuoles and polyphosphate content.
5. **What are Much's granules?**
   These are Gram-positive and non-acid-fast form of tubercle bacilli. Much (1907) demonstrated the presence of granules in cold abscess pus where there was no evidence of acid-fast bacilli.
6. **What is the role of malachite green in LJ medium?**
   Malachite green inhibits the growth of organisms other than mycobacteria and provides a colour contrast against which colonies of mycobacteria can be easily seen.
7. **Why prolonged incubation of LJ medium is required to culture *M. tuberculosis*?**
   The average generation time of tubercle bacilli is about 14–15 hours, prolonged incubation is, therefore, necessary.
8. **Describe the colonies of *M. tuberculosis* on LJ medium.**
   Colonies of *M. tuberculosis* on LJ medium are rough, tough and buff.
9. **What is the effect of sodium pyruvate in LJ medium on the growth of mycobacteria?**
   Sodium pyruvate improves the growth of both *M. tuberculosis* and *M. bovis*.
10. **What is the effect of glycerol (in LJ medium) on the growth of mycobacteria?**
    Growth of human tubercle bacillus is enhanced by 0.75% glycerol, but glycerol at this concentration is inhibitory to *M. bovis*. However, 0.5% glycerol still improves the growth of *M. tuberculosis* but generally does not inhibit the growth of *M. bovis*.
11. **Name disinfectants which can destroy tubercle bacilli.**
    Tincture of iodine and 80% ethanol
12. **How do you interpret positive Mantoux test?**
    0.1 ml of purified protein derivative (PPD) containing 5 IU is injected intracutaneously into the skin of the volar aspect of the forearm. The site of inoculation is palpated 72 hours later. The development of an area of palpable, firm induration 10 mm or more in diameter is recorded as positive.
13. **Enumerate conditions in which tuberculin test is false negative.**
    - Early tuberculosis
    - Miliary/advanced tuberculosis
    - Measles
    - Sarcoidosis
    - Lymphoreticular malignancy
    - Defective CMI
14. **Enumerate conditions in which BCG vaccination is contraindicated.**
    - Tuberculosis
    - AIDS
    - Measles
    - Pertussis
    - Eczema
    - Tuberculin positive individuals
    - Patients on steroids
15. **Name mycobacteria causing skin ulcers.**
    - *M. ulcerans*
    - *M. balnei*

16. **How many tubercle bacilli can be detected by culture on LJ medium?**
It can detect as few as 10–100 bacilli per ml.

17. **What happens when CSF is taken from a case of tuberculous meningitis and allowed to stand?**
CSF from tuberculous meningitis often develops a spider web clot on standing.

18. **What do you mean by positive tuberculin test?**
A positive tuberculin test indicates hypersensitivity to tuberculoprotein denoting clinical or subclinical infection with tubercle bacillus, or BCG immunization.

19. **Which *Mycobacterium* has not been cultured in vitro?**
Mycobacterium leprae

20. **Which *Mycobacterium* causes swimming pool granuloma?**
M. marinum

21. **What do you mean by the term 'MOTT'?**
Mycobacteria other than tubercle bacilli that normally exist as saprophytes of soil and water and occasionally cause opportunistic disease in man resembling tuberculosis are known as atypical, environmental, opportunistic tuberculoid mycobacteria or mycobacteria other than tubercle (MOTT) bacilli.

Practical

30

Diagnostic Approach to Anaerobes

Anaerobes are organisms that do not require oxygen for life and reproduction. In addition, oxygen's direct toxic effect may prohibit the growth of these organisms in environments in which oxygen is present. Anaerobes outnumber aerobes at mucosal surfaces. These heavily colonized surfaces are the usual portals of entry into the tissues and blood stream for endogenous anaerobes. Factors that commonly predispose the human body to anaerobic infections include trauma of mucous membranes or skin, vascular stasis, tissue necrosis, and decrease in the redox potential of tissue. Certain hints suggest that a given specimen is likely to contain anaerobic bacteria:

- Foul odour
- Gas in specimen
- Black discolouration of blood containing exudates, these exudates may fluoresce red under ultraviolet light involving pigmented *Bacteroides*
- Presence of 'sulphur granules' in discharges (actinomycosis)
- Infection secondary to human or animal bite
- Location of infection in proximity to mucosal surface
- Infection persists despite aminoglycoside therapy

Specimen collection

Collection of specimens with swab should be discouraged because they dry out and also because they expose anaerobes, if present, to ambient oxygen. Specimens collected with needle and syringe are better for anaerobic bacteriology than those collected with swab.

The specimens acceptable for anaerobic culture and the collection methods that avoid contamination with normal flora are listed in Table 30.1.

Specimen transport

Regardless of the type of specimen submitted for anaerobic bacteriology, it must be transported and processed as rapidly as possible and with minimum exposure to oxygen. Transporting specimens within a needle and syringe assembly is no longer acceptable because of the hazard of accidental skin puncture. The aspirate should be injected into some type of oxygen-free transport tube or vial, preferably one containing a prereduced anaerobically sterilized (PRAS) transport medium such as the Hungate tube.

Tissue specimens collected by biopsy or at autopsy from usually sterile sites are acceptable specimens for

Table 30.1. Acceptable specimens for anaerobic bacteriology

Source	*Recommended methods of collection*
Localized abscesses	Needle and syringe aspiration of closed abscesses
Sinus tracts or draining wounds	Aspiration with syringe and small plastic catheter introduced as deeply as possible through decontaminated skin orifice
Deep tissue or bone	Specimens obtained during surgery form depth of wound or underlying bone lesion
Central nervous system	Cerebrospinal fluid, aspirated abscess material, tissue from biopsy or autopsy
Dental/ENT specimens	Aspirated abscess material, biopsied tissue

anaerobic culture. Small pieces of tissue can be placed in oxygen-free transport tubes or vials containing PRAS medium to keep the tissue moist. Larger tissues may be transported in bags or pouches containing an oxygen-free atmosphere to prevent exposure to oxygen enroute to the laboratory.

Processing of specimens

Ideally, once a specimen arrives in the laboratory, it is placed immediately in an anaerobic chamber to prevent further exposure of specimens to oxygen. All anaerobic chambers contain a catalyst, dessicant, H_2 gas (5–10%), CO_2 gas (5–10%), N_2 gas (80–90%) and an indicator.

- Macroscopic examination of the specimen
- Microscopic examination of the specimen
- Inoculation of non-selective, selective, enriched and liquid media
- Anaerobic incubation of inoculated media

Macroscopic examination of specimen

The specimen is inspected for characteristics that include:

- Foul odour
- Black discharge or black necrotic tissue
- Sulphur granules
- Brick red fluorescence

Microscopic examination of specimen

This examination always includes a Gram stain. This helps in preliminary identification of organisms and initiation of appropriate antibiotic therapy. This also helps in selection of the media to be inoculated.

Inoculation of solid and liquid media

The ideal media for use in the culture of anaerobes are those that have been freshly prepared or stored under anaerobic conditions from the time they were made. Anaerobes have special nutritional requirements for vitamin K, haemin and yeast extract, and all primary isolation media for anaerobes should contain these three ingredients. Liquid media soon become aerobic unless a reducing agent is added. Liquid media should be prereduced by holding in a boiling water-bath for 10 minutes to drive off dissolved oxygen, then quickly cooled to 37°C just before use. Different media are inoculated depending upon the organisms suspected.

Anaerobic incubation of inoculated media

Inoculated plates are incubated anaerobically at 37°C for at least 48 hours, and reincubated for another 2–4 days to allow slow-growing organisms to form colonies. The most conmmon choices for anaerobic incubation systems are anaerobic chambers, anaerobic jars, and anaerobic bags or pouches.

Anaerobic jars

The most widely used anaerobic jar is the McIntosh-Fildes' anaerobic jar. Inoculated culture plates are placed inside the jar after creating anaerobic condition. The gasPak is now the method of choice for preparing anaerobic jar. The gasPak is commercially available as disposable envelope containing chemicals which generate hydrogen and carbon dioxide on the addition of water. After the inoculated plates are kept in the jar, the gasPak envelope witn water added, is placed inside and the lid is screwed tight. Hydrogen and carbon dioxide are liberated and the presence of a cold catalyst in the envelope permits the combination of hydrogen and oxygen to produce an anaerobic environment. Methylene blue indicator is used for verifying the anaerobic conditions in the jar. When it is placed in an anaerobic environment it is reduced from its coloured oxidized form to a colourless reduced leuco-compound.

Anaerobic bags or pouches

These bags are available commercially and one or two inoculated plates are placed into a bag and an oxygen removal system is activated and the bag is sealed and incubated. Plates can be examined for growth without removing the plates from bag, thus without exposing the colonies to oxygen. But as with anaerobic jar, plates must be removed from the bags in order to work with the colonies at the bench. These bags are also useful for the transportation of biopsy specimens for anaerobic cultures.

Anaerobic chamber

This is an ideal anaerobic incubation system, which provides oxygen-free environment for inoculating media and incubating cultures. Identification and susceptibility tests can also be performed in anaerobic chambers.

Discussion

1. **Define obligate or strict anaerobes.**
   Obligate anaerobes may be defined as microorganisms that cannot multiply in the presence of more than 0.5% O_2 and are killed by exposure to air within a few minutes.

2. **Define moderate anaerobes.**
   Moderate anaerobes may be defined as microorganisms that cannot tolerate an atmosphere containing more than 2–8% O_2.

3. **Define aerotolerant anaerobes.**

   Aerotolerant anaerobes may be defined as microorganisms that are capable of growing in an atmosphere containing molecular oxygen but grow best in an anaerobic environment.

4. **Classify nonsporing anaerobes.**

   (i) **Cocci**

   Gram-positive
   - *Peptococcus*
   - *Peptostreptococcus*
   - *Sporosarcina*

   Gram-negative
   - *Veillonella*

   (ii) **Bacilli**

   Gram-positive
   - *Lactobacillus*
   - *Bifidobacterium*
   - *Propionibacterium*
   - *Actinomyces*

   Gram-negative
   - *Bacteroides*
   - *Fusobacterium*
   - *Leptotrichia*

   (iii) **Spirochaetes**
   - *Treponema*
   - *Borellia*

5. **Enumerate conditions that predispose a patient to anaerobic infections.**
   - Human or animal bite
   - Road-side accidents
   - Aspiration of oral contents into the lungs after vomiting
   - Tooth extraction or oral surgery
   - Gastrointestinal or genital tract surgery

6. **Which catalyst is used in McIntosh-Fildes' anaerobic jar?**

   Alumina pellets coated with palladium

7. **What is the role of catalyst in anaerobic jar?**

   It converts hydrogen and oxygen into water.

8. **Enumerate chemical and biological indicators for the anaerobic jar.**

   Chemical indicator : Methylene blue

   Biological indicator : A strict anaerobe such as *Clostridium tetani* or *Bacteroides fragilis*, and a strict aerobe, such as *Pseudomonas aeruginosa.*

9. **Define cancrum oris or noma.**

   Noma is a fulminant gangrenous infection of the oral and facial tissues that occurs in severely malnourished and debilitated patients. It begins as a necrotic ulcer in the gingiva of the mandible and caused by oral anaerobes, especially fusospirochetal organisms.

Practical 31

Clostridium

Introduction

Clostridia are anaerobic, Gram-positive, spore-bearing bacilli. Spores are refractile, oval or spherical and usually wider than the parent cell. They may be terminal, subterminal or central in the cell. Most clostridia possess flagella and are motile except *C. perfringens.*

Clostridium perfringens (Clostridium welchii)

Morphology

They are large, Gram-positive, spore-bearing bacilli measuring 4–6 × 1 μm with straight parallel sides and truncated or slightly rounded ends. They occur singly, in pairs or in small bundles. They are non-motile and form capsule in animal body. Spores are oval, subterminal or central and non-bulging (Fig. 31.1A). They are formed under natural conditions e.g. in the bowel. They are only rarely seen in direct smears from wounds or cultures but can be demonstrated on growth in special media such as Ellner's medium.

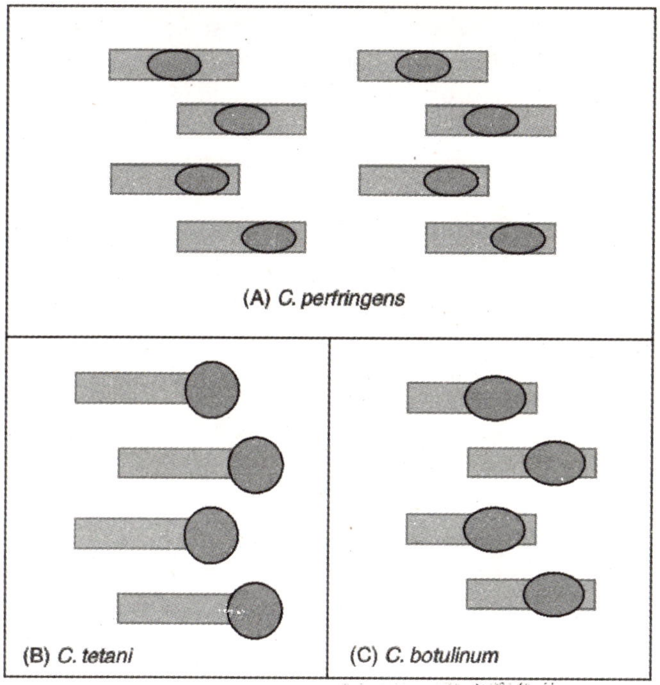

Fig. 31.1. (A) *Clostridium perfringens*, (B) *C. tetani*, (C) *C. botulinum.*

Cultural characteristics

It is an anaerobe, but can grow under microaerophilic conditions. Optimum temperature for growth is 37°C. It grows best on media containing carbohydrate such as glucose blood agar and forms two main types of colonies. One is round, 2–4 mm in diameter, smooth, regular, convex, amorphous, greyish-yellow and slightly opaque. Other is umbonate with an opaque brownish centre and a lighter, translucent, radially striated periphery with a crenated edge. On horse blood agar, colonies are usually surrounded by a zone of β-haemolysis and commonly also by an outer wider zone of incomplete haemolysis owing to the action of θ and α toxins respectively (double zone haemolysis) (Colour Plate VI, Fig. 35).

Biochemical reactions

It is actively saccharolytic. When grown in cooked meat broth (CMB), they rapidly produce acid and gas but they do not digest the meat. The culture may have a slightly sour smell and the meat is often reddened. It ferments glucose, maltose, sucrose, lactose and starch with the production of acid and gas. In litmus milk medium, it ferments lactose and produce acid and gas. The acid clots the milk and gas breaks up the clot resulting in *stormy clot reaction*. Production of acid is also indicated by change in the colour of the litmus from blue to red. The culture has sour butyric acid odour. It is indole negative, MR positive, VP negative and H_2S positive.

Gelatin is liquefied but coagulated serum is usually not liquefied. It produces phospholipase-C which gives opalescence around the colonies on egg-yolk containing medium.

Nagler's reaction

This is a useful test for the rapid detection of *C. perfringens* in clinical specimens. Several clostridia like *C. perfringens, C. novyi, C. bifermentans* and some vibrios, produce phospholipase enzyme that gives rise to opalescence in both human serum and egg-yolk containing media. The reaction produced by *C. perfringens* is specifically neutralized by *C. perfringens* antitoxin, but serologically related phospholipases of *C. bifermentans* and *C. sordellii* and some other phospholipases are also neutralized.

For rapid detection of *C. perfringens*, a culture plate containing 6% agar, 5% peptic digest of sheep blood and 20% human serum or 5% egg-yolk is prepared. The plate is dried. On one half of the plate, 2–3 drops of *C. perfringens* antitoxin are spread and allowed to dry. The plate is then inoculated with the test organism or the exudate under study and incubated anaerobically at 37°C for 18 hours. On the section containing no antitoxin, *C. perfringens* colonies show surrounding zone of opalescence i.e. Nagler's reaction whereas colonies of the remainder half of the plate show no change (Fig. 31.2). Neomycin sulphate may be added to this medium to inhibit aerobic spore-forming organisms and coliforms.

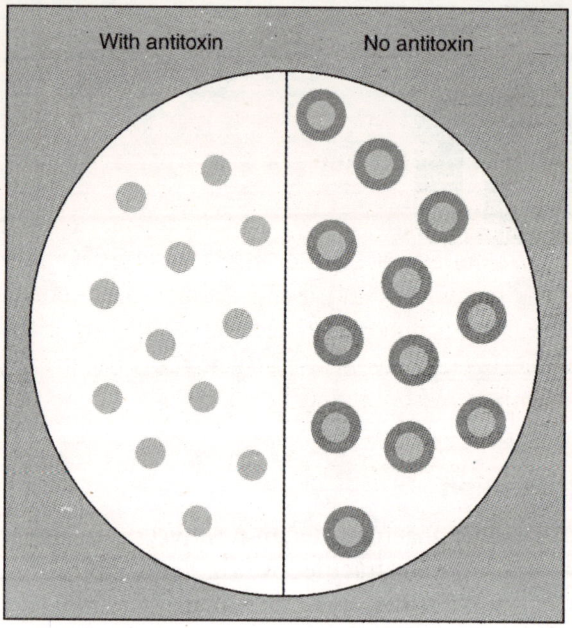

Fig. 31.2. Nagler's reaction.

Clostridium tetani

Morphology

C. tetani is a slender, Gram-positive bacillus, 2–5 × 0.4–0.5 μm with rounded ends. It tends to be pleomorphic and filamentous. It is non-capsulated and motile by peritrichate flagella. The spores are spherical, terminal and twice the diameter of vegetative cells giving them typical drumstick appearance (Fig. 31.1B). The spores do not take up the Gram stain and appear as colourless round structures.

Cultural characteristics

C. tetani is an obligate anaerobe. The optimum temperature and pH for its growth are 37°C and 7.4 respectively. It can grow well on ordinary media, but its growth is improved by the addition of blood or serum and in CMB. Colonies on solid media are irregularly round, 2–5 mm in diameter with fine branching projections. Some strains form colonies with thicker, translucent, yellow brown centre and thin, translucent, colourless periphery. Isolated colonies of *C. tetani* may not be obtained because of the tendency of the organism to swarm over the surface of the medium. However, non-motile variants may produce isolated colonies.

Horse blood agar

On this medium, the colonies of *C. tetani* are surrounded by a zone of α-haemolysis, which subsequently develops into β-haemolysis owing to the production of an oxygen-labile haemolysin known as tetanolysin.

Egg-yolk agar

On this medium, it does not produce opalescence or pearly layer.

CMB

It grows well in CMB. The meat is not digested but shows slight blackening on prolonged incubation (slightly proteolytic).

Biochemical reactions

It has no saccharolytic activity.

Indole	+
MR	–
VP	–

H_2S	–
Nitrate reduction	–
Gelatin	Slowly liquefied

Clostridium botulinum

Morphology

C. botulinum is a straight or slightly curved Gram-positive bacillus with rounded ends. It measures about 5 × 1 μm in size. It is non-capsulated and motile by peritrichate flagella. It produces heat-resistant spores that are oval, subterminal and bulging (Fig. 31.1C).

Cultural characteristics

It is an obligate anaerobe. Optimum temperature for growth is 35°C, but some strains can grow and produce toxin at 1–5°C. It can grow well on routine culture media. Surface colonies are large, irregular, smooth, semitransparent with fimbriate border. On horse blood agar, all strains except those of type G are β-haemolytic. All types except G produce opalescence and a pearly effect on egg-yolk agar.

Biochemical reactions

Indole	–
Gelatinase	+
Lecithinase-C activity	–

All strains except G (A,B,C,D,E,F) have lipase activity and ferment glucose, maltose and sucrose with the production of acid. They do not ferment lactose.

Discussion

1. **Name clostridia which are non-motile.**
   - *C. perfringens*
   - *C. tetani* type VI
2. **Enumerate predominantly saccharolytic clostridia.**
   - *C. perfringens*
   - *C. septicum*
   - *C. novyi*
3. **Enumerate predominantly proteolytic clostridia.**
   - *C. sporogenes*
   - *C. histolyticum*
   - *C. bifermentans*
4. **Enumerate clostridia which are obligate anaerobes.**
   - *C. septicum*
   - *C. novyi*
   - *C. tetani*
5. **Why *C. perfringens* is also called as *C. welchii*?**
   This is after the name of the scientist, Welch who first described this bacterium in detail.
6. **Which *Clostridium* produces 'stormy clot reaction' in litmus milk medium?**
   C. perfringens
7. **What do you mean by double zone haemolysis or target haemolysis?**
   After overnight incubation on horse blood agar, colonies of *C. perfringens* are surrounded by a narrow zone of β-haemolysis due to theta (θ) toxin and also by an outer wider zone of incomplete haemolysis due to alpha (α) toxin. This is known as double zone haemolysis.
8. **Enumerate organisms which produce phospholipase enzyme and hence Nagler's reaction.**
   - *C. perfringens*
   - *C. novyi*
   - *C. bifermentans*
   - Some vibrios
   - Some aerobic spore-formers
9. **Enumerate clostridia causing gas gangrene.**
   - *C. perfringens*
   - *C. novyi*
   - *C. septicum*
   - *C. histolyticum*
   - *C. sordellii*
10. **Name clostridia which produce swarming on solid media.**
    - *C. tetani*
    - *C. septicum*
11. **Which *Clostridium* is responsible for pseudomembranous colitis and antibiotic-associated diarrhoea?**
    C. difficile
12. **Name clostridia which show typical drumstick appearance.**
    - *C. tetani*
    - *C. tetanomorphum*
    - *C. sphenoides*

13. **Which toxin is considered as the most toxic substance known to mankind?**
Botulinum toxin

14. **Does the food poisoning caused by *C. botulinum* lead to diarrhoea or constipation ?**
Constipation

15. **What is the mechanism of action of botulinum toxin?**
It is a neurotoxin which apparently acts by inhibiting the release of acetylcholine from the motor nerve endings of the parasympathetic system.

16. **Why tetanus patients are isolated in the hospital?**
The reason for isolation is to protect them from noise and light which may provoke the convulsions. Tetanus patients are hardly ever infectious, and person to person transmission does not occur at all.

17. **Does an attack of tetanus confer immunity?**
No, an attack of the disease does not confer immunity. Second attacks of tetanus have been recorded.

18. **What is the therapeutic role of botulinum toxin?**
Botulinum toxin is given as intramuscular injection to treat strabismus.

19. **How many *C. perfringens* are carried in faeces of healthy individuals?**
10^3–10^4 organisms per gram of faeces are carried in healthy individuals.

20. **Name selective medium for the isolation of *Clostridium perfringens.***
Willis and Hobbs medium

21. **What is the immunization schedule for individuals who have not been immunized for tetanus in infancy?**
The immunization should be carried out with 3 spaced intramuscular injections. The intervals recommended are 6–8 weeks between the first and second injections and 4–6 months between the second and third and booster doses every 10 years.

Practical 32

Escherichia Coli

Morphology

It is a Gram-negative, non-capsulated bacillus measuring 1–3 μm × 0.4–0.7 μm in size. Most (about 80%) strains are motile by peritrichous flagella. The fimbriae are present on 80% of the strains. In most of the strains, these are of type I, i.e. haemagglutinating and mannose-sensitive and are found in both motile and non-motile strains. A few strains, especially those from extra intestinal infections, possess polysaccharide capsule and many other form abundant loose slime when grown on sugar-containing medium at 15–20°C.

Cultural characteristics

It is an aerobe and facultative anaerobe. Optimum temperature for its growth is 37°C (range 10–45°C). It can grow on ordinary media like nutrient agar.

Nutrient agar

Colonies are large (2–3 mm in diameter), circular, low convex, colourless, opaque or partially translucent after 18 hours incubation at 37°C.

MacConkey agar

Colonies are red or pink in colour due to lactose fermentation (Colour Plate VII, Fig. 36).

Deoxycholate citrate agar (DCA)

The growth is partially or totally inhibited by sodium citrate and sodium thiosulphate. Colonies that form are small, pink and opaque.

Blood agar

Colonies of some strains of *Escherichia coli* are surrounded by a complete zone of haemolysis.

Biochemical reactions

Test	Result
Indole	+
MR	+
VP	–
Citrate utilization	–
Urease test	–
H_2S production	–
Phenylalanine deaminase test	–
Gelatin liquefaction	–
Malonate utilization	–
Acid and gas from	
glucose	+
mannitol	+
maltose	+
lactose	+
sucrose	+

Indole production and fermentation of sugars takes place both at 37°C and 44°C. Variants of *E. coli* that utilize citrate have been isolated. The citrate-utilizing ability has been shown to be controlled by a transmissible plasmid. Similarly, H_2S positive variants of *E. coli* have also been described in which the ability to produce H_2S is controlled by a transmissible plasmid.

Discussion

1. **Enumerate various toxins produced by *E. coli*.**
   - Enterotoxins
     Heat-labile toxin
     Heat-stable toxin
   - Haemolysin
   - Verotoxin

2. **Which organism is the commonest cause of urinary tract infection (UTI)?**

   E. coli

3. **Define urinary tract infection.**

   Urinary tract infection may be defined as the presence of bacteria undergoing multiplication in urine within the urinary drainage system.

4. **What do you mean by Kass concept of significant bacteriuria?**

   Kass gave a criterion of active bacterial infection of urinary tract according to which a count exceeding 10^5 organisms/ml denotes significant bacteriuria and indicates active UTI.

5. **Why there is relative infrequency of UTI in males?**

   Relative infrequency of UTI in males is due to following factors:
   - Long urethra
   - Bactericidal activity of prostatic fluid

6. **Which enterotoxin of *E. coli* is antigenically related to cholera toxin?**

   Heat-labile toxin-I (LT-I) is antigenically related to cholera toxin.

7. **Which toxin of *E. coli* is identical to Shiga toxin?**

   Verotoxin 1 (VT 1) (phage encoded cytotoxin)is identical to the Shiga toxin.

8. **Enumerate various pathogenic lesions produced by *E. coli.***
   - Urinary tract infection
   - Diarrhoea and dysentery
   - Pyogenic infections
   - Septicaemia

9. **Enumerate various groups of *E. coli* causing diarrhoeal diseases.**
   - Enteropathogenic *E. coli* (EPEC)
   - Enterotoxigenic *E. coli* (ETEC)
   - Enteroinvasive *E. coli* (EIEC)
   - Enteroaggregative *E. coli* (EAEC)
   - Verotoxigenic *E. coli* (VTEC)

10. **Which strains of *E. coli* are responsible for traveller's diarrhoea?**

    Enterotoxigenic *E. coli*

11. **What do you mean by Sereny test?**

    Sereny test is used to detect enteroinvasive *E. coli* (EIEC). The organism is instilled into the conjuctival sac of guinea-pig and examined after 72 hours for the production of keratoconjuctivitis.

12. **What is haemolytic uraemic syndrome (HUS)?**

    HUS is characterized by acute renal failure, microangiopathic haemolytic anaemia and thrombocytopenia.

13. **Which strains of *E. coli* are responsible for HUS?**

    Verotoxigenic *E. coli* (VTEC).

Practical 33

Klebsiella

Morphology

They are Gram-negative, non-sporing, non-motile bacilli, 1–2 μm long and 0.5–0.8 μm wide with parallel or bulging sides and slightly pointed or rounded ends. They occur either in end to end pairs or are arranged singly. Freshly isolated strains possess a well defined polysaccharide capsule. In the Gram-stained smears, capsule appears as an empty halo around the bacterium. Some extracellular polysaccharide is also secreted from the bacteria as loose soluble slime, accumulation of which gives mucoid appearance to the colonies. Non-capsulated and non-slime forming mutants appear from time to time. They form small and non-mucoid colonies. Klebsiellae do not have flagella but most strains possess fimbriae of one or more of three types, 1, 3 and 6.

Cultural characteristics

Klebsiellae grow well on ordinary media in a temperature range of 12–43°C with optimum growth at 37°C. On MacConkey agar, the colonies typically appear large, mucoid and red (Colour Plate VI, Fig. 37). However, some strains are not mucoid.

Biochemical reactions

Biochemical reactions of different subspecies of *Klebsiella pneumoniae* and *K. oxytoca* are given in Table 33.1.

Discussion

1. **Enumerate various subspecies of *K. pneumoniae*.**
   - *Aerogenes*
   - *Ozaenae*
   - *Pneumoniae*
   - *Rhinoscleromatis*
2. **Which subspecies of *K. pneumoniae* is most frequently isolated?**
   Subsp. *aerogenes* is most frequentely isolated.

Table 33.1. Differentiation of species and subspecies of *Klebsiella*

	***K. pneumoniae* subspecies**				***K. oxytoca***
	aerogenes	*ozaenae*	*pneumoniae*	*rhinoscleromatis*	
Indole	–	–	–	–	+
MR	–	+	+	+	v
VP	+	–	–	–	v
Citrate	+	v	+	–	+
Urease	+	–	+	–	+
Lactose (acid production)	+	+	+	–	+
ONPG	+	+	+	–	+

3. **Name indole positive species of *Klebsiella*.**

   K. oxytoca

4. **Which serotypes are most frequently associated with human respiratory tract infection?**

   Types 1–6

5. **Enumerate pathogenic lesions caused by klebsiellae.**
   - Hospital associated (nosocomial) urinary tract infection
   - Wound and burn infection
   - Bronchopneumonia
   - Septicaemia
   - Meningitis
   - Diarrhoea

6. **Which *Klebsiella* is associated with atrophic rhinitis?**

   K. pneumoniae subsp. *ozaenae*

7. **What is the other name given to *K. pneumoniae*?**

   Friedlander's bacillus

Practical 34

Proteus

Tribe Proteeae, in the family Enterobacteriaceae, comprises three genera: *Proteus, Morganella* and *Providencia*. The tribe has a unique ability to oxidatively deaminate amino acids to the corresponding keto acids and ammonia. It is tested by growing the organism in a medium containing phenylalanine, from which phenylpyruvic acid is formed (PPA test). Genus *Proteus* has four species: *P. mirabilis, P. vulgaris, P. myxofaciens* and *P. penneri.*

Morphology

They are Gram-negative coccobacilli, 1–3 μm long and 0.6 μm wide. In young cultures, most of them are long (up to 80 μm) curved and filamentous. They may be arranged singly, in pairs or in short chains. They are actively motile by peritrichous flagella. However, non-flagellate and non-motile variants are also encountered. They also possess more than one type of fimbriae.

Cultural characteristics

They can grow on ordinary media like nutrient agar and culture emits characteristic putrefactive (fishy or seminal) odour. *P. mirabilis* and *P. vulgaris* possess the ability to swarm (spread) on solid media (Colour Plate VII, Fig. 38). Swarming of *Proteus* appears to be due to vigorous motility of the organism. Non-motile variants do not swarm. Swarming does not occur on MacConkey agar on which smooth, colourless colonies are formed.

Dienes phenomenon

When two identical strains of *Proteus* are inoculated at different points of the same culture plate, without any swarming inhibiting substance, the resulting swarms of growth coalesce without signs of demarcation. When, however, two different strains of *Proteus* species are inoculated, the spreading films of growth fail to coalesce and remain separated by a narrow but easily visible furrow. This is known as Dienes phenomenon. It has been used to determine the identity or non-identity of various strains of *Proteus*.

Biochemical reactions

All species of *Proteus* produce acid from glucose and no acid from lactose, mannose, mannitol, inositol, sorbitol and arabinose. They do not utilize malonate and are positive for nitrate reduction test. Differentiation of four species of *Proteus* is given in Table 34.1.

Table 34.1. Differentiation of four species of *Proteus*

	Proteus			
	mirabilis	*vulgaris*	*penneri*	*myxofaciens*
Swarming on solid media	+	+	–	–
Indole	–	+	–	–
MR	+	+	+	+
VP	v	–	–	+
Citrate utilization	v	v	–	v
Phenylalanine deaminase test	+	+	+	+
Urease production	+	+	+	+
H_2S production	+	+	–	+

Discussion

1. **Briefly describe the types of swarming exhibited by *Proteus*.**

   Continuous swarming : Swarming growth on a culture plate appears as a uniform film of growth extending over the whole plate.

   Discontinuous swarming: Swarming growth on a culture plate appears as a series of concentric circles of growth around the point of inoculation.

2. **Enumerate various agents which can inhibit swarming of *Proteus*.**
   - Increasing the concentration of agar in the medium from 1–2% to 6%.
   - Incorporating chloral hydrate (1 in 500), sodium azide (1 in 500), alcohol (5–6%) or boric acid (1 in 100) in the medium.
   - Addition of bile salts in the medium.

3. **Name one unique test for tribe Proteeae.**

   PPA test

4. **Enumerate four species of genus *Proteus*.**
   - *P. mirabilis*
   - *P. vulgaris*
   - *P. myxofaciens*
   - *P. penneri*

5. **Which species of *Proteus* is indole positive?**

   Proteus vulgaris

6. **Which species of *Proteus* shows swarming on solid nutrient media?**
   - *P. vulgaris*
   - *P. mirabilis*

7. **What is the characteristic odour of *Proteus* culture?**

   Fishy or seminal odour

8. **What is the use of Dienes phenomenon?**

   Dienes phenomenon is used to determine the identity or non-identity of various strains of *Proteus.*

9. **Which species of *Proteus* is most frequently isolated from clinical specimens?**

   P. mirabilis

10. **Why urinary tract infection caused by *Proteus* is more serious than that caused by coliform bacteria?**

    Proteus produces urease which liberates ammonia from urea. Ammonia inactivates complement, damages renal epithelium and makes the urine alkaline. The alkaline conditions lead to the precipitation of phosphates and the formation of calculi in the urinary tract. It may also lead to hyperammonaemic encephalopathy and coma.

11. **What do you understand by the term *Proteus*?**

    Proteus means pleomorphism and the name is after the Greek God *Proteus* who could assume any shape.

Practical 35

Shigella

The genus *Shigella* is closely related to the genus *Escherichia* and belongs to the tribe Escherichieae. *Shigella* species, however, are not members of the normal gastrointestinal flora, and all *Shigella* species can cause bacillary dysentery. Genus *Shigella* has four species: *Shigella dysenteriae, Shigella flexneri, Shigella sonnei* and *Shigella boydii.*

Morphology

Shigellae are non-motile, non-flagellate, non-sporing, non-capsulated, Gram-negative bacilli measuring 2–4 × 0.6 μm. *S. flexneri*, with the exception of serotype 6 and some strains of other serotypes, possess fimbriae of type 1. Other species of *Shigella* do not possess fimbriae.

Cultural characteristics

They are aerobes and facultative anaerobes, growing within a temperature range of 10–40°C and pH of 7.4. They can grow on ordinary media.

Nutrient agar

On nutrient agar or blood agar, colonies are 2–3 mm in diameter, circular, convex, smooth, greyish or colourless and translucent. Colonies of *S. sonnei* are slightly larger and more opaque than those of other shigellae.

MacConkey agar

Colonies on this medium are colourless due to the absence of lactose fermentation. However, colonies of *S. sonnei*, a late lactose-fermenter, become pink when incubation is prolonged beyond 24 hours.

Deoxycholate citrate agar (DCA)

This is a selective medium for isolation of shigellae from faeces. Colonies on this medium are smaller (1–1.5 mm in diameter) and do not form a black centre. On prolonged incubation, colonies of *S. sonnei* form pink papillae due to late lactose fermentation.

Xylose lysine deoxycholate (XLD) agar

This is a better selective medium than DCA because it is less inhibitory to *S. dysenteriae* and *S. flexneri* than DCA. On this medium, colonies of *Shigella* are red and unlike those of most salmonellae, without black centres (Colour Plate VII, Fig. 39).

Salmonella-Shigella (SS) agar

This is a highly selective medium for the isolation of *Shigella* and *Salmonella*. Colonies of *Shigella* on this medium are colourless with no blackening (Colour Plate VII, Fig. 40).

Hektoen enteric (HE) agar

This is a useful direct plating medium for faecal specimens for the isolation of *Shigella* and *Salmonella.* Colonies of *Shigella* on this medium are green in colour (Colour Plate VII, Fig. 39).

Enrichment media

- *Selenite F broth* : Sodium selenite in this medium inhibits coliform bacilli while permitting shigellae and salmonellae to grow. Therefore, it is recommended for the isolation of these organisms from faeces.

- *Gram-negative (GN) broth* : Enrichment of faecal specimens in GN broth for 4–6 hours and then subculturing on HE or XLD agar is an optimal technique for recovery of *Shigella* species in suspected cases of bacillary dysentery.

Biochemical reactions

Indole	V
MR	+
VP	–
Citrate utilization	–
Urease	–
H_2S production	–

All shigellae produce acid from glucose and with the exception of *S. dysenteriae*, from mannitol. *S. dysenteriae* serotype 1, *S. flexneri* serotype 6 and *S. sonnei* are always indole negative. *S. sonnei* is a late lactose-fermenter and forms ornithine decarboxylase. With the exception of *S. dysenteriae* serotype 1, many strains of *S. dysenteriae* serotypes 3, 4, 6 and 9, *S. flexneri* serotype 4a, and *S. boydii* serotype 13; shigellae produce catalase.

Discussion

1. **Who isolated the first member of the genus *Shigella*?**
   Japanese microbiologist Kiyoshi Shiga isolated the first member of the genus. It was then called *S. shigae* and is now known as *S. dysenteriae* serotype 1.
2. **Enumerate four species of *Shigella*.**
   - *S. dysenteriae*
   - *S. flexneri*
   - *S. sonnei*
   - *S. boydii*
3. **Which species of *Shigella* is more resistant to adverse environmental conditions as compared to other species?**
   S. sonnei
4. **What is the infective dose of shigellae?**
   The infective dose is small between 10–100 organisms.
5. **Which *Shigella* species is most pathogenic?**
   S. dysenteriae
6. **Enumerate toxins produced by *S. dysenteriae* serotype 1.**
   - Exotoxin (acts as enterotoxin and neurotoxin)
   - Verotoxin – VT1 and VT2
   - Endotoxin
7. **Which is the most predominant species of *Shigella* in India?**
   S. flexneri
8. **Which is the most prevalent species of *Shigella* in the United State?**
   S. sonnei
9. **Which species of *Shigella* produce mild infection?**
   S. sonnei
10. **Enumerate complications produced by *S. dysenteriae* serotype 1.**
    - Haemolytic uraemic syndrome
    - Intussusception
    - Parotitis
    - Toxic neuritis
    - Arthritis
11. **How will you differentiate ulcers of *Shigella* dysentery from those of amoebic ulcers?**
    The ulcers of the bacillary dysentery are much shallower than amoebic ulcers. The intervening mucosa is inflammed and oedematous in bacillary dysentery. Thus there is diffuse involvement, unlike the amoebic dysentery in which the mucosa in between the ulcerative lesions is healthy.
12. **What is the incubation period of *Shigella* dysentery.**
    It is usually 2–3 days, but may be as short as 12 hours.

Practical 36

Salmonella

Morphology

Salmonellae are Gram-negative, non-sporing, non-acid-fast, non-capsulated bacilli measuring 2–4 × 0.6 μm. Most strains are motile by means of peritrichous flagella except *S.* Gallinarun and *S.* Pullorum which are non-motile. Most strains of most serotypes produce type 1 fimbriae. Most strains of *S.* Paratyphi A and a few strains of *S.* Paratyphi B, *S.* Typhi and *S.* Typhimurium fail to produce fimbriae.

Cultural characteristics

Salmonellae are aerobes and facultative anaerobes, growing within a temperature range of 15–45°C (optimum temperature 37° C). They can grow on ordinary media.

Nutrient agar or blood agar

Colonies on these media are 2–3 mm in diameter, greyish-white, circular, moist, convex and translucent. Rough (R) strains form opaque and granular colonies with irregular surface. They have a hydrophobic surface and tend to autoagglutinate. Due to the production of loose polysaccharide slime, many strains of *S.* Paratyphi B and a few of other serotypes form large mucoid colonies.

MacConkey agar

Colonies are 1–3 mm in diameter and pale yellow or colourless due to absence of lactose fermentation (Colour Plate VII, Fig. 41).

Brilliant green MacConkey agar

This is a selective medium for the isolation of salmonellae from feaces. Salmonellae produce pale green translucent colonies. However, *S.* Typhi does not grow well on this medium.

Deoxycholate citrate agar

Colonies are similar to or slightly smaller in size than those on MacConkey agar. After 48 hours incubation, the colonies may develop a black centre.

Wilson and Blair's brilliant-green bismuth sulphite agar medium

On this medium, *S.* Typhi and *S.* Paratyphi B form small (about 1 mm in diameter) black colonies (Colour Plate VII, Fig. 42). This is due to the reduction of sulphite to sulphide. Due to the production of hydrogen sulphide, the colonies of *S.* Typhi are surrounded by a metallic sheen. Brilliant green inhibits the gowth of *Escherichia coli*, *Proteus* and other commensal enterobacteria.

Xylose lysine deoxycholate agar

Most strains of *Salmonella* produce red colonies with black centres (Colour Plate VII, Fig. 42) and H_2S negative serotypes of *Salmonella* produce red colonies without black centres.

Salmonella–Shigella agar

Colonies of *Salmonella* are colourless with black centres (Colour Plate VII, Fig. 43).

Hektoen enteric agar

Colonies of *Salmonella* are blue green with black centres due to H_2S production (Colour Plate VII, Fig. 43).

Enrichment media

- *Tetrathionate broth* : It enriches salmonellae and sometimes shigellae, but permits the growth of *Proteus.*

- *Brilliant green tetrathionate broth* : Brilliant green in tetrathionate broth inhibits the growth of *Proteus*, thus makes it more selective for the growth of salmonellae. But it is also inhibitory, to some extent, to *S.* Typhi and shigellae.
- *Selenite F broth* : It is an excellent enrichment medium for the isolation of *S.* Typhi and *S.* Dublin, but some salmonellae e.g. *S.* Paratyphi A and *S.* Choleraesuis and some shigellae may fail to grow in this medium.

Biochemical reactions

Test	Result	Remarks
Indole	–	
MR	+	
VP	–	
Citrate utilization	+	(except *S.* Typhi and *S.* Paratyphi A)
H_2S production	+	(except strains of *S.* Paratyphi A and *S.* Choleraesuis)
Urease	–	
Phenylalanine deaminase test	–	
Acid and gas from		
glucose	+	*S.* Typhi and *S.* Gallinarum form acid only
maltose	+	
mannitol	+	
sorbitol	+	
lactose	–	
sucrose	–	

Discussion

1. **Name non-motile serotypes of *Salmonella*.**
   S. Gallinarum and *S.* Pullorum
2. **Name selective media for isolation of *Salmonella*.**
   Wilson and Blair's brilliant-green bismuth sulphite agar, deoxycholate citrate agar, xylose lysine deoxycholate agar and *Salmonella-Shigella* agar
3. **Enumerate pathogenic lesions produced by *Salmonella*.**
   - Enteric fever or typhoid fever
   - Gastroenteritis
   - Septicaemia
4. **Enumerate complications of typhoid fever.**
   - Intestinal perforation
   - Haemorrhage
   - Circulatory collapse
   - Other complications include cholecystitis, arthritis, haemolytic anaemia, peripheral neuritis and rarely osteomyelitis.
5. **What do you mean by rose spots?**
   Rose spots are often found on the front of the chest during the second or third week of typhoid fever. These are 2–4 mm in diameter, slightly raised discrete irregular macules. They are seldom noticeable in dark-skinned patients.
6. **When should you perform faecal culture for isolation of salmonellae in patient of typhoid fever?**
   Faecal culture should be done between third to fifth week of illness.
7. **What is the advantage of clot culture over blood culture in diagnosis of typhoid fever?**
   - Clot culture yields a higher rate of isolation than blood culture as the bactericidal action of the serum is obviated.
   - Sample of serum also becomes available for Widal test.
8. **Name one oral vaccine for typhoid fever.**
   S. Typhi (Ty 21a)
9. **Which serotype of *Salmonella* is associated with septicaemia?**
   Salmonella septicaemia is commonly caused by *S.* Choleraesuis.
10. **Enumerate serotypes of *Salmonella* causing gastroenteritis.**
    S. Typhimurium, *S.* Enteritidis, *S.* Newport and *S.* Dublin
11. **Name killed vaccine of *Salmonella*.**
    TAB Vaccine
12. **Which specimen is most appropriate for culture of *Salmonella* in first week of enteric fever?**
    Blood
13. **Which medium is used for blood culture in case of enteric fever?**
    Bile broth
14. **Which specimens are important for detection of carriers of *Salmonella*?**
    Faeces and bile
15. **For determining the serotype of infecting organism, detection of which agglutinin is more important in Widal test?**
    'H' agglutinin

16. **What are the typical clinical features of typhoid fever?**
The typical clinical features of typhoid fever are step-ladder pyrexia, with relative bradycardia and tox-aemia.

17. **What do you mean by term 'Typhoid Mary'?**
Mary Mallon (Typhoid Mary) was a typhoid carrier, a New York cook who, over a period of 15 years, caused at least seven outbreaks affecting over 200 persons.

Practical 37

Pseudomonas

The genus *Pseudomonas* belongs to the family Pseudomonadaceae which contains over 200 species. Majority of them are free-living, occurring as saprophytes in soil and water. Human disease has been caused by *P. aeruginosa, P. fluorescens, P. putida* and *P. stutzeri.*

Pseudomonas aeruginosa

Morphology

It is a slender, Gram-negative bacillus, 1.5–3.0 µm × 0.5 µm, arranged singly, in pairs or short chains. It is non-sporing, non-capsulated, though mucoid strains may sometime occur and usually motile by one or two polar flagella.

Cultural characteristics

It is strict aerobe and grows well on ordinary media. It can grow over a temperature range of 5–42°C, the optimum temperature being 37°C.

Nutrient agar

After aerobic incubation on nutrient agar at 37°C for 24 hours, the colonies are large, 2–3 mm in diameter, smooth, translucent, irregularly round (Colour Plate VII, Fig. 44) and emit a characteristic fruity odour. Mucoid strains often produce copious amount of an extracellular polysaccharide on agar culture.

MacConkey agar

It produces non-lactose-fermenting colonies.

Blood agar

Many strains are haemolytic on blood agar.

***P. aeruginosa* produces at least 4 distinct pigments:**

1. *Pyocyanin* : It is bluish-green phenazine pigment soluble in chloroform and water. It diffuses into the surrounding medium. This pigment is not produced by other species of this genus, therefore, its detection is diagnostic of *P. aeruginosa.*
2. *Pyoverdin (fluorescein)* : It is soluble in water but not in chloroform. It imparts a yellowish tinge to the cultures.
3. *Pyorubin* : It is bright red water soluble pigment. It is a phenazine pigment that is insoluble in chloroform.
4. *Pyomelanin* : It is brown to black pigment and its production is uncommon.

Biochemical reactions

The metabolism of *P. aeruginosa* is oxidative and nonfermentative.

Test	Result
Catalase	+
Oxidase	+
Indole	–
MR	–
VP	–
H_2S production	–
Nitrate reduction to N_2 gas	+
Arginine dihydrolase	+
Gelatinase	+

Discussion

1. **Why does culture of *Pseudomonas aeruginosa* emit a characteristic fruity odour?**
   This is due to the production of aminoacetophenone from tryptophan.

2. **Enumerate pigments produced by *P. aeruginosa.***
   - Pyocyanin
   - Pyoverdin
   - Pyorubin
   - pyomelanin
3. **What is the chemical nature of pyocyanin produced by *P. aeruginosa* ?**

   It is a phenazine pigment.
4. **Does pigment produced by *P. aeruginosa* diffuse into the medium?**

   Yes
5. **Name one pigment of *P. aeruginosa* which is soluble in chloroform.**

   Pyocyanin
6. **Name one pigment which is produced only by *P. aeruginosa.***

   Pyocyanin
7. **Name one disinfectant to which *Pseudomonas* is sensitive.**

   It is sensitive to 2% aqueous alkaline solution of glutaraldehyde (cidex).
8. **Name selective medium used for isolation of *P. aeruginosa.***

   Cetrimide agar
9. **Enumerate common infections caused by *P. aeruginosa.***
   - Urinary tract infection
   - Meningitis
   - Necrotizing pneumonia
   - Septicaemia
   - Wound and burn infections
   - Chronic otitis media and otitis externa
10. **Why *P. aeruginosa* is dominant bacterium in mixed infections?**

    P. aeruginosa produces pyocyanin pigment, which inhibits the growth of many other bacteria.
11. **Why *P. aeruginosa* is frequently responsible for nosocomial infections?**

    P. aeruginosa is important causative agent of nosocomial infections due to following reasons:
    - It is resistant to commonly used antibiotics and antiseptics.
    - It can survive and multiply even with minimal nutrients, if moisture is available.
    - It can contaminate equipment such as respirators, endoscopes and articles such as bed pans and medicines such as lotions, ointments and eye drops.
12. **Name one species of *Pseudomonas* which can grow at 42°C.**

    P. aeruginosa
13. **Enumerate tests to identify non-pigment producing *P. aeruginosa.***
    - Oxidative metabolism of sugars
    - Positive oxidase test
    - Ability to reduce nitrate to nitrogen gas
    - Growth at 42°C
14. **Name pigments enhancing media of *Pseudomonas.***
    - *Pseudomonas* isolation agar
    - King's medium (A and B)

Practical

38

Vibrio

The genus *Vibrio* belongs to family Vibrionaceae. Genus *Vibrio* has at least 33 well defined species. The most important pathogens of man are *V. cholerae, V. parahaemolyticus* and *V. vulnificus.*

Vibrio cholerae

Morphology

These are short, curved or comma-shaped rods with rounded or pointed ends and 1.5–2.5 × 0.5–0.8 μm in size. S forms or spirals may be seen due to two or more cells lying end to end (Fig. 38.1). In old cultures, they are frequently highly pleomorphic. They show vigorous darting motility which is mediated by a single polar flagellum.

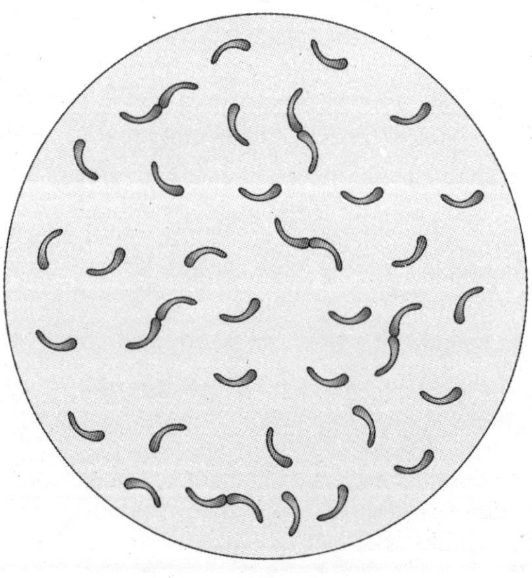

Fig. 38.1. *Vibrio cholerae.*

They are Gram-negative, non-sporing, non-capsulated and non-acid-fast.

Cultural characteristics

V. cholerae is aerobe and facultative anaerobe, but under anaerobic conditions only scanty and slow growth is obtained. It grows within a temperature range of 16–40°C (optimum temperature 37°C). Growth occurs freely between pH 7.4 and 9.6 (optimum pH 8.2). *V. cholerae* is a non-halophilic vibrio. It cannot grow in media with a concentration of sodium chloride more than 5%. However, it can grow in media without any sodium chloride. On the other hand, halophilic vibrios like *V. parahaemolyticus* can grow in media containing 7–10% sodium chloride and cannot grow in media lacking it.

On nutrient agar, after overnight incubation at 37°C, the colonies are glistening translucent discs, 1–2 mm in diameter with bluish or greenish tinge in transmitted light. On MacConkey agar, they are smaller than those on nutrient agar and are colourless, but become reddish on prolonged incubation due to the late fermentation of lactose. On horse blood agar, classical biotype does not produce haemolysis although some strains produce greenish discolouration around individual colonies which later becomes clear due to haemodigestion. However, colonies of El Tor biotype are haemolytic.

In a gelatin stab, at first a white line of growth appears along the track of the inoculating wire. Liquefaction of gelatin begins at the top which spreads downwards in a funnel-shaped form (infundibuliform appearance) in 3 days at 22°C. In peptone water, this organism grows as a surface pellicle because of its affinity for oxygen. The surface pellicle becomes visible in 6–9 hours.

Special media

A number of special culture media have been employed for the cultivation of *V. cholerae*. They may be classified as under:

Transport (holding) media

- *Venkatraman-Ramakrishnan (VR) medium*
- *Cary-Blair medium*

Enrichment media

Alkaline peptone water (APW) : This medium contains 1% each of peptone and sodium chloride at pH 8.6. This is also an excellent transport medium. About 1g of the stool or a rectal swab should be placed into 10 ml of APW in a screw-capped bottle and transported to the laboratory. Subcultures on plating media should be done within 3–6 hours because other organisms can begin to overgrow after prolonged incubation.

Plating media

Alkaline bile salt agar (BSA) pH 8.2 : This is modified nutrient agar medium containing 0.5% sodium taurocholate. The colonies on BSA are similar to those on nutrient agar medium.

Monsur's gelatin taurocholate trypticase tellurite agar (GTTA) medium : This medium is useful for the isolation of cholera and other vibrios from faeces. After 24 hours incubation, vibrios produce small (1–2 mm) translucent colonies with greyish-black centre and a turbid halo, due to hydrolysis and denaturation of gelatin. After 48 hours incubation, colonies increase in size to 3–4 mm.

Thiosulphate-citrate-bile-sucrose (TCBS) agar : This is most commonly used selective plating medium for vibrios. This medium resembles DCA except that it contains sucrose instead of lactose. Sucrose-fermenting vibrios such as *V. cholerae* form yellow colonies and non-sucrose-fermenters such as *V. parahaemolyticus* blue green ones (Colour Plate VIII, Fig. 45).

Biochemical reactions

Catalase	+
Oxidase	+
Indole	+
MR	–
VP	+ (El Tor biotype)
Nitrate reduction	+
Acid from	
glucose	+
sucrose	+
mannitol	+
maltose	+
mannose	+
lactose	late lactose-fermenter
Gelatin liquefaction	+

Cholera red reaction

V. cholerae is strongly indole positive and reduces nitrates to nitrites. These two properties contribute to the 'cholera red reaction', the development of a red colour when concentrated sulphuric acid is added to a 4 day old culture at 37°C in peptone water. It is due to the formation of nitrosoindole which is red in colour.

Discussion

1. **Enumerate species of genus *Vibrio* which are pathogenic to man.**
   - *V. cholerae*
   - *V. parahaemolyticus*
   - *V. vulnificus*
2. **What is the characteristic motility of *V. cholerae*?**
   Darting motility
3. **How much sodium chloride concentration can be tolerated by *V. cholerae*?**
   V. cholerae can tolerate sodium chloride concentration up to 5%.
4. **What do you mean by term 'halophilic vibrios'?**
   Halophilic vibrios can grow in media containing 7–10% sodium chloride and cannot grow in media lacking it.
5. **Enumerate halophilic vibrios.**
   - *V. parahaemolyticus*
   - *V. vulnificus*
   - *V. alginolyticus*
6. **Which type of colonies are produced by *V. cholerae* on MacConkey agar?**
   Colonies are colourless after 24 hours incubation, but become reddish on prolonged incubation due to late fermentation of lactose.
7. **Name late lactose-fermenting organisms.**
   - *V. cholerae*
   - *Shigella sonnei*

8. **Which biotype of *V. cholerae* produces haemolysis on blood agar plate?**
El Tor biotype

9. **Enumerate transport media of *V. cholerae.***
   - Venkatraman-Ramakrishnan (VR) medium
   - Cary-Blair medium

10. **Why there is need of transport media for *V. cholerae?***
V. cholerae is quite sensitive to drying, exposure to sunlight and extreme changes in pH. It is also inhibited by normal intestinal flora. So if the cultures cannot be put up immediately, then the stool samples should be transported in transport media.

11. **What alternative can be used, if transport medium is not available?**
If a transport medium is not available, a 5 cm × 1.5 cm strip of thick blotting paper can be soaked in the faecal matter, then placed in a sealed plastic bag, and sent to the laboratory.

12. **What should be the pH of alkaline peptone water (APW)?**
The pH of APW should be 8.6.

13. **What is the advantage of high pH of APW?**
High pH of the medium suppresses the growth of many commensal intestinal bacteria while permitting uninhibited growth of *V. cholerae.*

14. **Which organism shows cholera red reaction?**
V. cholerae

15. **How many biotypes of *V. cholerae* are there?**
Two biotypes: classical and El Tor

16. **Differentiate between classical and El Tor biotypes of *V. cholerae.***

Property	*Biotype*	
	Classical	*El Tor*
Voges-Proskauer test	–	+
Agglutination of fowl RBCs	–	+
Haemolysis of sheep RBCs	–	+
Sensitivity to:		
• Polymyxin B	+	–
• Mukerjee's group IV phage	+	–
• Basu and Mukerjee's group V phage	–	+

17. **Why vibrios do not survive in grossly contaminated water, such as the Ganges water in India?**
This is perhaps due to the presence of a large number of vibriophages in this water.

18. **Which biotype of *V. cholerae* is hardier?**
El Tor

19. **How many serogroups of *V. cholerae* are there?**
There are 193 serogroups or serovars which depend upon 193 different 'O' antigens.

20. **Name choleragenic serogroups of *V. cholerae.***
Two recognized choleragenic serogroups of *V. cholerae* are: serogroups O1 and O139.

21. **What do you mean by non-O1, non-O139 vibrios?**
The serogroups (O2 to O138 and O140 to O193) are referred to as non-O1, non-O139, vibrios. Before the advent of serogroup O139, serogroups O2 to O138 were also known as non-cholera vibrios or non-agglutinable (NAC) vibrios as they are not agglutinated by O1 antisera.

22. **How many subtypes of O1 serogroup of *V. cholerae* are there?**
O1 serogroup can be further subdivided into three subtypes: Ogawa, Inaba and Hikojima.

23. **What is the characteristic of stool in *V. cholerae* infection?**
The cholera stool is typically a colourless watery fluid with flakes of mucus and hence called rice water stool.

24. **Describe the mechanism of action of cholera toxin.**
It consists of subunit A and B. The A is active subunit and B is binding subunit. The subunit A stimulates cell bound adenylate cyclase. This, in turn, converts ATP to cyclic adenosine monophosphate (CAMP) in the gut epithelial cells (enterocytes). This causes an irreversible hypersecretion of electrolytes and water out of the cell and into the lumen of the intestine.

25. **Which biotype of *V. cholerae* is responsible for mild and asymptomatic infections?**
El Tor

26. **Which species of *Vibrio* is responsible for food poisoning?**
V. parahaemolyticus

Practical

39

Spirochaetes

Treponema

Treponemes are slender spirochaetes with fine spirals and pointed ends. Some of them are pathogenic for man, while others occur as commensals in mouth and genitalia. *Treponema* species pathogenic for man include the causative agents of venereal syphilis (*T. pallidum*) and non-venereal treponematoses: yaws (*T. pertenue*), endemic syphilis (*T. endemicum*) and pinta (*T. carateum*).

Treponema pallidum

Morphology

It is a thin, delicate, long, motile, flexible organism which is twisted spirally around its long axis. It is 6–14 µm long. Its width is 0.13 µm in dried state, but is about 0.2 µm in the wet living state, which is just great enough for resolution with the light microscope. It has 6–12 coils which are remarkably evenly disposed at 1 µm intervals and the amplitude of spirals is 1–1.5 µm. They have tapering ends. It is actively motile exhibiting flexion and extension, translatory and corkscrew-like motility. As the spirochaete moves across the dark-field of the microscope, it often displays a characteristic tendency to bend at right angle near its midpoint. These secondary curves appear and disappear but its primary spirals remain unchanged.

T. pallidum cannot be seen under the light microscope in wet films. Its morphology and motility can be seen under the dark-ground microscope (Fig. 39.1). It cannot be stained by simple aniline dyes or by Gram's method. By prolonged Giemsa staining it stains pale pink. It can be stained by silver impregnation methods. Fontana's method is useful for staining films and Levaditi's method for tissue sections. By immunoflorescence method, treponemes can be detected in tissues and body fluids.

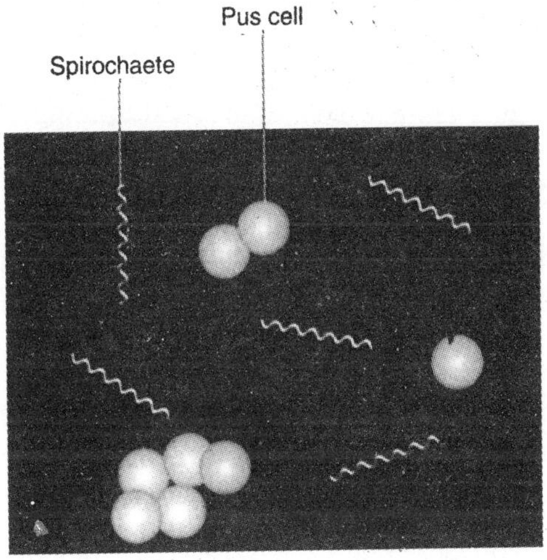

Fig. 39.1. Dark-ground illumination preparation of serous exudate from primary syphilitic chancre.

Ultrastructurally, *T. pallidum* possesses usually three but occasionally four endoflagella attached subterminally at each end of the cell and extend towards the opposite pole between outer membrane and peptidoglycan layer and cytoplasmic fibrils that run the length of the organism internal to cytoplasmic membrane.

Cultivation

Pathogenic treponemes cannot be cultivated in artificial media and are maintained by subculture in susceptible animals. Nichols strain of *T. pallidum* has been maintained, in rabbit testis, for several decades by serial testicular passages since it was isolated in 1913 from CSF of a patient with neurosyphilis. The mean generation time for growth, in vivo, in the rabbit testis appears to be 30 hours. It can be maintained, in vitro, for 1–6 days, using maintenance medium (Nelson medium) that contains rabbit serum, reducing agents, vitamins, cofactors, amino acids and salts. Eagle and McCoy cell culture medium supplemented with foetal bovine serum and reducing agents may also be used for the maintenance of the organism. Cultivable treponemes such as *T. phagedenis* (Reiter treponeme) and *T. refringens* are nonpathogenic. They can be grown under strictly anaerobic conditions in Smith-Noguchi medium or in digest broth enriched with serum.

Discussion

1. **Which type of motility is seen in *Treponema pallidum*?**

   T. pallidum is actively motile exhibiting flexion and extension, translatory and corkscrew-like motility. As the spirochaete moves across the dark-field of the microscope, it often displays a characteristic tendency to bend at right angle near its midpoint. The secondary curves appear and disappear but its primary spirals remain unchanged.

2. **Which disease is caused by *T. pallidum*?**

   T. pallidum causes syphilis.

3. **How can you prevent transfusion syphilis?**

   Transfusion syphilis can be prevented by storing blood for at least 5 days in the refrigerator before transfusion.

4. **Enumerate routes of transmission of syphilis.**
   - Sexual intercourse
   - Blood transfusion.
   - Congenital (mother-to-foetus)

5. **How many stages of syphilis are there?**

   There are four stages of syphilis :
   - Primary syphilis
   - Secondary syphilis
   - Latent syphilis
   - Tertiary syphilis

6. **Which type of chancre is produced in primary syphilis?**

   Hard chancre. It is also known as Hunterian chancre, after John Hunter who produced the lesion on himself experimentally.

7. **Which organs are involved in tertiary syphilis?**

   Tertiary syphilis involves following organs :
   - Heart and aorta
   - Joints
   - Central nervous system
   - Skin and mucous membranes

8. **Enumerate oral manifestations of congenital syphilis.**
   - Hutchinson's incisors
   - Mulberry molars
   - Gummatous lesions of palate, jaws and facial bones
   - Glossitis
   - Mucous patches
   - Fissures of corners of mouth

9. **In which stage of syphilis oral lesions may be present?**

   Oral lesions may be present in all the three stages of syphilis (primary, secondary and tertiary).

10. **What is the oral complication of tertiary syphilis?**

    Gumma may destroy palate, causing complete perforation.

11. **What is the first noticeable lesion in endemic syphilis (bejel)?**

    Intraoral mucous patch.

Practical 40

Oral Microbiology

Normal flora of the mouth

Normal flora or the microbiota refers to the population of microorganisms that inhabits skin and mucous membranes of normal healthy persons.

The normal microbial flora of the oral cavity is complex and consists of large number of species of bacteria, fungi and protozoa.Microbial flora varies qualitatively and quantitatively after tooth eruption, tooth extraction, artificial dentures, dental treatments (scaling , polishing, filling), the frequency and type of food ingested and antibiotics treatment.

The oral cavity may be considered as an ideal microbial incubator. It possesses an abundance of moisture, an excellent supply of various types of foods and differences in oxygen tension. Many aerobic, facultative and anaerobic organisms find conditions favourable for growth (Table 40.1)

At birth the mouth of the newborn is usually sterile. Within a few hours of the birth streptococci, of which *Streptococcus salivarius* is dominant, establish themselves in the mouth. During the first month of life, other species of streptococci, staphylococci, neisseriae, veillonellae, lactobacilli, *Actinomyces* and fusobacteria also colonize. Eruption of teeth provides hard surfaces in the oral cavity. These are colonized by *S. mutans*, *S. sanguis* and *Actinomyces viscosus*.

Dental plaque

Dental plaque is a soft, adherent dental deposit that forms as a result of bacterial colonization of the tooth surface. One gram of plaque contains approximately 2×10^{11} bacteria. In addition, plaque may also contain host cells such as epithelial cells, macrophages and leucocytes. Based on its position on the tooth surface, dental plaque is classified as supragingival, marginal and subgingival plaque.

Table 40.1. Bacterial flora of the oral cavity

Gram-positive cocci	*Gram negative cocci*	*Gram-positive bacilli*	*Gram-negative bacilli*
Streptococcus salivarius	*Neisseria* spp.	*Actinomyces israelii*	*Bacteroides* spp.
S. sanguis	*Veillonella* spp.	*A. viscosus*	*Treponema vincentii*
S. mutans		*A. naeslundii*	*T. denticola*
S. sorbinus		Lactobacilli	*T. refringens*
S. cricetus			*Porphyromonas gingivalis*
S. rattus			*Actinobacillus actinomycetemcomitans*
S. gordonii			*Fusobacterium* spp.
S. mitis			*Prevotella* spp.
S. milleri			*Capnocytophaga* spp.
Staphylococcus aureus			
S. epidermidis			
Micrococcus spp.			
Peptostreptococcus spp.			

If the plaque is left undisturbed then calcium and phosphate ions derived from saliva may become deposited within deeper layers of dental plaque and form a calcified mass of plaque, termed **calculus.** Calculus, therefore, consists of mineralized bacterial plaque. It can form extensive deposits around the teeth. Calculus per se is not directly implicated in disease but acts as a nidus for further plaque accumulation.

Dental caries

Dental caries is a chronic endogenous infection caused by the normal oral flora. The carious lesion is the result of demineralization of enamel- and later of dentine-by acids produced by plaque microorganisms as they metabolize dietary carbohydrates. However, the initial process of enamel demineralization is usually followed by remineralization, and cavitation occurs when the former process overtakes the latter.

For dental caries to develop from a plaque, the appropriate microorganisms need to be present on susceptible tooth surface, with access to suitable substrates (such as trapped food, salivary glycoproteins) for an adequate time. Initially, cocci predominate in the plaque and produce extracellular matrix. This matrix is then colonized by other bacteria including filamentous bacteria and anaerobes. Organic acids and enzymes produced by the microorganisms cause decalcification, proteolysis, and slow, progressive decay of the tooth, starting with the covering enamel.

When the surface layer of enamel has been lost, the infection invariably progresses to dentine, with the pulp becoming firstly inflamed and then necrotic.

The rate of caries has dramatically dropped in countries such as the United States , where improved oral hygiene and fluoridation of the drinking water has become a standard practice. Fluoride incorporates into the crystalline structure of enamel, forming fluoropatite, and contributes to resistance to degradation by bacterial acids.

Periodontal diseases

Periodontal diseases can be defined as disorders of supporting structures of the teeth, including the gingival, periodontal ligament and supporting alveolar bone. Periodontal disease can be broadly categorized into **gingivitis** and **periodontitis**.

Acute necrotizing ulcerative gingivitis

It is commonly associated with poor and neglected oral hygiene, malnutrition, heavy smoking, emotional stress, primary herpetic gingivostomatitis and infection with human immunodeficiency virus. The disease is a specific, anaerobic, polymicrobial infection mainly due to the combined activity of fusobacteria (*Fusobacterium nucleatum*) and oral spirochaetes (*Treponema* spp.). It may also be caused by *Prevotella intermedia, Veillonella* and streptococci.

Chronic gingivitis

Chronic gingivitis is characterized by gingival redness, oedema, bleeding, changes in contour, and loss of tissue adaptation to the teeth. It is caused by prolonged exposure of host tissue to a non-specific mixture of gingival plaque organisms. These includes *Streptococcus sanguis, S. millleri, Actinomyces israelii, A. naeslundii, Prevotella intermedia, Capnocytophaga* spp., *Fusobacterium nucleatum* and *Veillonella* spp.

Chronic periodontitis (formerly adult periodontitis)

Periodontitis refers to an inflammatory process that affects the supporting structures of the teeth : periodontal ligaments, alveolar bone and cementum. With progression, periodontitis can lead to serious sequelae, including the loosening and eventual loss of teeth.

Microorganisms implicated in chronic periodontitis are *Actinobacillus actinomycetemcomitans, Porphyromonas gingivalis, Prevotella intermedia, Fusobacterium nucleatum, Bacteroides forsythus, Selenomonas* spp., *Capnocytophaga* spp. and *Treponema* spp.

Localized and generalized aggressive periodontitis

The disease is more common in West Africans and Asians. It appears around puberty. It has rapid progress with active and quiscent periods. It is relatively common in girls and case clusters are usually seen in families.

In the localized variant the incisors and/or first permanent molars in both jaws are affected for unknown reason. Later other teeth may be involved, producing the appearance of generalized alveolar bone loss. In generalized variant of the disease many areas may be involved in a similar manner.

Aggressive periodontitis is caused by *Actinobacillus actinomycetemcomitans, capnocytophaga* spp., *Porphyromonas gingivalis* and *Prevotella intermedia.* This disease may be associated with cellular immune or genetic defects.

Dentoalveolar abscess

Dentoalveolar infection may be defined as pyogenic infections associated with the teeth and surrounding supporting structure, such as the peridontium and the alveolar bone. A dentoalveolar abscess usually develops by the extension of the initial carious lesion into dentine, and spread of bacteria to the pulp via the dentinal tubules.

Dentoalveolar abscess may be caused by obligate anaerobes and facultative anaerobes. Pus should be collected by needle aspiration, or in a sterile container after external incision. Both anaerobic and aerobic cultures are done using conventional methods and isolates identified.

Discussion

1. **Define dental plaque.**
   Dental plaque may be defined as the soft deposits that form the biofilm adhering to the tooth surface or other hard surfaces in the oral cavity, including removable restorations.
2. **What is the composition of dental plaque?**
   It consists of dense masses of a variety of microorganisms from the normal flora, proteins from the saliva, and desquamated epithelial cells.
3. **How many bacteria are present in a gram of plaque?**
   One gram of plaque contains approximately 2×10^{11} bacteria.
4. **Enumerate bacteria which colonize the dental plaque.**
   - *Actinomyces viscosus*
   - *Streptococcus sanguis*
   - *Streptococcus mutans*
   - *Prevotella intermedia*
   - *P. loescheii*
   - *Fusobacterium nucleatum*
   - *Porphyromonas gingivalis*
5. **Define calculus.**
   Calcium and phosphate ions deposition within deeper layers of dental plaque to form a calcified mass of plaque is called as calculus.
6. **What is role of pyrophosphate compounds in toothpastes?**
   Pyrophosphate compounds adsorb excess calcium ions, thus reducing intraplaque mineral deposition.
7. **What is the role of fluoridation of drinking water?**
   Fluoride incorporates into the crystalline structure of enamel, forming fluoropatite, and contributes to resistance to degradation by bacterial acids.
8. **Which is the most common cause of tooth loss in children and young adults ?**
   Dental caries
9. **Which is the most common cause of tooth loss after the age of 35?**
   Chronic periodontitis
10. **Enumerate cariogenic streptococci.**
    - *Streptococcus mutans*
    - *S. sorbinus*
    - *S. cricetus*
    - *S. rattus*
11. **What are the various strategies to prevent dental caries?**
    Dental caries may be prevented by:
    - Stopping or reducing between meal consumption of carbohydrates
    - Making the tooth structure less soluble to acid attack by using fluorides
    - Using sealants to protect pits and fissures
    - Reducing cariogenic flora by mechanical cleansing, antimicrobial therapy and immunization
    - Replacement of cariogenic bacteria by genetically engineered mutans streptococci
12. **Enumerate causative agents of dentoalveolar abscess.**
    Obligate anaerobes :
    - *Prevotella intermedia*
    - *P. melaninogenicus*
    - *Porphyromonas gingivalis*
    - *Fusobacterium nucleatum*
    - *Peptostreptococcus* spp.

    Facultative anaerobes
    - *Streptococcus milleri*
    - *Actinomyces* spp.
13. **Which microorganisms are the predominant supragingival bacteria?**
    Streptococci
14. **Define dental caries.**
    Dental caries may be defined as localized destruction of the tissues of the tooth by bacterial fermentation of dietary carbohydrates.
15. **How do you recognize initial caries lesion?**
    Initial caries lesion is recognized by 'White spot' created by the demineralization of enamel.

16. **Which form of periodontitis is by far the most prevalent globally?**
Chronic periodontitis

17. **Enumerate causative agents of acute necrotizing ulcerative gingivitis.**
    - *Fusobacterium nucleatum*
    - *Treponema* spp.

18. **What are the key factors in the development of dental caries?**
    - Plaque bacteria
    - Host (susceptible tooth surface and saliva)
    - Diet (fermentable carbohydrates)

19. **Enumerate protozoa normally present in the oral cavity.**
    - *Entamoeba gingivalis*
    - *Trichomonas tenax*

20. **Enumerate fungi normally present in the oral cavity.**
    - *Candida albicans*
    - *C. dubliniensis*
    - *C. glabrata*
    - *C. tropicalis*
    - C. *krusei*

21. **By which year of life, the oral microbial flora of the child resembles that of adult?**
By the first year of life.

22. **What are the major causes of tooth loss?**
    - Dental caries
    - Chronic periodontitis

23. **Which tissues of the tooth are affected in chronic periodontitis?**
    - Periodontal ligament
    - Alveolar bone

24. **Enumerate plaque-related diseases.**
    - Dental caries
    - Gingivitis
    - Periodontitis

25. **Where does plaque accumulates in oral cavity?**
Plaque accumulates in non-self-cleansing areas of teeth such as pits and fissures, along the gingival margins and between the teeth.

26. **Enumerate initiators of plaque formation.**
    - *Streptococcus mutans*
    - *Streptococcus sanguis*
    - *Actinomyces* spp.

27. **How many bacterial species are present in mature dental plaque?**
Three hundred to 400.

28. **What is the prime element of oral hygiene?**
Removal of plaque is the prime element.

29. **Which substances help in removal of plaque?**
    - Tooth paste
    - Mouthrinse additives
        - phenolic compounds
        - essential oils
        - triclosan
        - fluorides
        - herbal extracts
        - quaternary ammonium compounds

30. **Which organisms are considered to be the main initiators of dental caries?**
Streptococci, chiefly *S. mutans* and *S. sorbinus*

31. **Enumerate complications of dental caries.**
    - Pulpitis
    - Necrosis of pulp
    - Periapical abscess
    - Periapical granuloma
    - Cellulitis
    - Osteomyelitis
    - Septic thrombophlebitis

32. **Is gingivitis a reversible disease?**
Yes

33. **Is periodontitis a reversible disease?**
No. The lost alveolar bone and periodontal ligament do not regenerate with cessation of the inflammation.

34. **Which organism is mainly associated with localized aggressive periodontitis?**
Actinobacillus actinomycetemcomitans

35. **Is acute necrotizing periodontal disease painless condition?**
No, acute necrotizing periodontal disease is painful. There is rapid ulceration of the interdental areas of the gingiva, resulting in destruction of the interdental papillae.

36. **Enumerate antibacterial substances present in saliva.**
    - Lysozyme
    - Lactoperoxidase
    - Secretory IgA

37. **Which dye is used to stain tissues of oral cavity?**
Erythrocin

38. **Which disease is called as trench mouth or vincent's angina?**
Acute necrotizing ulcerative gingivitis

39. **Define Ludwig's angina.**
Ludwig's angina is a rapidly spreading, life-threatening cellulitis of the sublingual and submandibular spaces that usually starts in an infected lower molar.

40. **How much fluoride ingestion can result in enamel discoloration?**
Daily ingestion of more than 1.5 mg fluoride can result in enamel discoloration.

41. **Which systemic diseases are associated with enamel hypoplasia?**
    - Hypoparathyroidism
    - Celiac diseases
    - Vitamin D- resistant rickets or disturbted calcium phosphate metabolism
    - Premature birth

42. **Which antibiotic should be avoided in pregnancy and in Infancy?**
Tetracycline. It can cause permanent discoloration of teeth and enamel hypoplasia.

43. **Enumerate oral infections causing halitosis.**
    - Acute primary herpetic gingivostomatitis
    - Acute necrotizing ulcerative gingivitis
    - Periodontal diseases
    - Caries

PART–5

Mycology

Contents

Practical 41

Laboratory Diagnosis of Mycoses

Introduction

Fungi are a group of non-motile eukaryotic organisms which are saprophytes, parasites or commensals. Infection caused by fungus is known as mycosis. Successful laboratory diagnosis of mycoses is dependent not only upon the mycologic expertise of the clinical laboratory workers but also heavily upon the quality of the specimens provided for laboratory analysis. Specimens for the diagnosis of mycoses include:

- *Superficial mycoses* – skin, nail, hair, wet swab or scrapings from mucous membrane
- *Subcutaneous mycoses* – pus, exudates, grains and biopsies
- *Systemic mycoses* – tissue biopsy, blood, sputum, cerebrospinal fluid, bone marrow aspirate, fluids and urine

Causative agents of mycoses can be identified by following methods:

Direct microscopic examination of specimens

Although the Gram stain performed in the routine microbiology laboratory often gives the first evidence of infection with yeasts, other direct stains give more specific information concerning a mold infection. The types of direct examination used in identification of fungal infection include wet preparation such as KOH preparation, KOH with calcofluor white, India ink and tissue stains such as periodic acid-Schiff (PAS) stain, Gomori's methenamine silver (GMS) stain, Giemsa stain and haematoxylin and eosin (H&E) stain.

KOH preparation

A 10–20% solution of KOH is useful for detecting fungal elements in skin, hair, nails and tissues. In this procedure, KOH is mixed in equal proportions with the specimen on a slide and the specimen material is teased with two inoculating needles. A cover-slip is placed over it and heated gently. Preparation with KOH clears the tissue and cellular debris from all types of clinical specimens without damaging the fungal cells. This clearing process requires only 5–10 minutes, after which one can observe the fungal morphology as well as the pigment of the fungal cell wall under a phase-contrast or bright-field microscope, using low-power followed by high-power objectives.

KOH with calcofluor white

A drop of 0.1% calcofluor white solution can be added to the KOH preparation prior to placing cover-slip over it. Calcofluor white binds to polysaccharide present in the chitin of the fungus or to cellulose. Fungal elements fluoresce apple green or blue-white, depending on the combination of filters used. The actual fungal structure must be seen before a positive preparation is reported.

India ink

India ink preparations may be used for detecting encapsulated yeast *Cryptococcus neoformans* in cerebrospinal fluid (CSF). A drop of India ink is mixed with a drop of centrifuged deposit of CSF, and the preparation is examined under high power. With this negative stain, budding yeast surrounded by a large clear area against a dark background is presumptive evidence of *C. neoformans*. White blood cells and other artifacts may resemble encapsulated organisms, therefore, careful examination is necessary.

Tissue stains

The diagnosis of fungal diseases should preferably be established on the basis of histopathological evidence combined with cultural evidence, because detection of fungi in tissue and confirmation of tissue invasion are required in diagnosing many opportunistic fungal infections. For example, isolation of common fungi such as *Aspergillus, Penicillium,* and *Rhizopus* species from sputum does not establish pulmonary infection by these fungi unless there is also histopathological evidence. Moreover, fixed histopathologic specimens often may be the only available material for diagnosis, and certain mycoses e.g. rhinosporidiosis, lobomycosis and *Pneumocystis carinii* infections can only be diagnosed by histologic studies since growth conditions of the fungi causing these infections have not been defined.

Culture

Relatively few types of standard media are needed for primary isolation of fungi. These include Sabouraud's dextrose agar (SDA), SDA with antibiotics, and brain-heart infusion (BHI) agar with blood and antibiotics. The pH of Emmons' modification of SDA is close to neutral and is more efficient for primary isolation than the original formulation. The antimicrobials usually included in SDA with antibiotics are chloramphenicol and gentamicin to inhibit bacterial growth and cycloheximide to inhibit saprophytic fungi. Special media may be used for isolation and to help rapid identification when the identity of a particular fungus is strongly suspected, for example, *C. neoformans* develops black colonies on bird seed agar.

Discussion

1. **Define the term fungi.**

   Fungi are a group of non-motile eukaryotic organisms which exist as saprophytes, parasites or commensals.

2. **What are dimorphic fungi?**

   Fungi that have two morphologic forms such as a mold and a yeast, which develop under different growth conditions e.g., *Histoplasma capsulatum* forms hyphae in vitro and yeast in tissues.

3. **Enumerate dimorphic fungi.**
   - *Histoplasma capsulatum*
   - *Sporothrix schenkii*
   - *Blastomyces dermatitidis*
   - *Coccidioides immitis*
   - *Paracoccidioides brasiliensis*
   - *Penicillium marneffei*

4. **What percentage of KOH is used for detecting fungal elements in keratinized tissues?**

   A 10–20% solution of KOH is used.

5. **Why cycloheximide is added to SDA medium?**

   Cyloheximide is added to inhibit saprophytic fungi.

6. **Why test tube agar slants are preferred for isolation of fungi as compared to agar plates?**

   Test tube agar slants are preferred because of the following reasons:
   - There are less chances of contamination.
   - They are more resistant to desiccation during protracted incubation.
   - They require less space.

7. **What precautions should be taken while using test tube agar slants?**
   - The culture tube should be large enough (2 × 15 cm) to provide a wide surface area for growth.
   - The screw caps should be left loosened during incubation to permit an adequate supply of oxygen or use sterile cotton plugs.

Practical 42

Candida Albicans

Introduction

Candida albicans is an oval or spherical budding yeast cell 3–5 μm in diameter. It produces pseudohyphae when the buds continue to grow but fail to detach, producing chains of elongated cells that are pinched or constricted at the septation between cells. It also can produce true hyphae. The yeast is a common commensal of the gastrointestinal tract, mucous membranes and skin. Since *Candida* is normally present on skin and mucosa, therefore, it is significant only when it is present in large numbers. In addition, presence of pseudohyphae indicates colonization. Gram-stained smears from lesions, exudates and skin and nail scrapings show budding Gram-positive yeast cells and pseudohyphae.

Candida albicans is the commonest cause of candidiasis (moniliasis). Candidiasis is an opportunistic endogenous infection. Predisposing factors for candidiasis are AIDS, diabetes mellitus, neutropaenia and prolonged administration of antimicrobial agents.

Cultural characteristics

Sabouraud's dextrose agar (SDA)

C. albicans grows well on SDA. Cream-coloured, smooth, pasty colonies appear in 1–2 days at 25–37°C (Colour Plate VIII, Fig. 46). Lactophenol cotton blue (LCB) preparation and Gram-stained smears show budding yeast cells and pseudohyphae (Colour Plate VIII, Fig. 47).

Corn meal agar

C. albicans produces large spherical chlamydospores which may be intercalary, terminal or sessile.

Test for presumptive Identification of *C. albicans*

Germ tube test

A germ tube is a filamentous outgrowth from a yeast cell. The filament lacks a constriction at the point of origin which differentiate it from the pseudohyphae.

Discussion

1. **Is *Candida albicans* a yeast or yeast-like?**
   It is yeast-like.
2. **Enumerate few tests for the identification of *Candida albicans*.**
   Two simple tests for the identification of *C. albicans* are:
   - Germ tube test
   - Chlamydospores formation on corn meal agar
3. **Enumerate *Candida* spp. which are positive for germ tube test.**
   - *C. albicans*
   - *C. dubiliensis*
4. **Enumerate lesions produced by *C. albicans*.**
   - *Mucocutaneous lesions* : Oral thrush, vulvovaginitis, conjuctivitis, balanitis and keratitis.
   - *Skin and nail infections* : Paronychia, infection of the skin at moist sites and napkin dermatitis in infants.
   - *Systemic candidiasis* : It may lead to urinary candidiasis, pulmonary candidiasis, hepatobiliary candidiasis, endocarditis, meningitis, arthritis, osteomyelitis and candidaemia.

5. **What is the significance of pseudohyphae of *C. albicans*?**

   Prensence of pseudohyphae indicates colonization.

6. **Enumerate oral manifestations of candidiasis.**
   - Thrush
   - Chronic oral candidiasis
   - Denture stomatitis
   - Chronic hypertrophic candidiasis
   - Chronic mucocutaneous candidiasis
   - Angular stomatitis
   - Circumoral candidal dermatitis

7. **Define Thrush.**

   Thrush is pseudomembranous candidiasis. The lesions are soft, white, slightly elevated plaques most frequently occuring on the palate, gingiva and floor of the mouth.

8. **What is the composition of candidal plaque?**

   The plaque consists chiefly of tangled masses of fungal hyphae with intermingled desquamated epithelial, keratin, fibrin, necrotic debris, leucocytes and bacteria.

9. **Which fungus produce oral lesions similar to those of candidiasis or thrush?**

   Geotrichum candidum

10. **Enumerate predisposing factors of thrush.**
    - Immunocompromised patients
    - Patients on long term antibiotic therapy
    - Neonates

Practical 43

Cryptococcus Neoformans

Introduction

Cryptococcus neoformans is a true yeast. It causes cryptococcosis, a sporadic or opportunistic yeast mycosis usually affecting the lungs, brain and meninges and occasionally other parts of the body.

Direct microscopy

India ink or nigrosin

The direct microscopy of CSF, mixed with a drop of India ink or nigrosin shows round budding yeast cells, 4–10 μm in diameter. The organisms are surrounded by a wide refractile gelatinous capsule that may be twice the size of the yeast cells. In India ink preparation, it appears as a clear halo around the yeast cells (Colour Plate I, Fig. 7).

Gram staining

In cryptococcal meningitis, the yeasts are often detected in a Gram-stained preparation of CSF sediment. They are Gram-positive but stain poorly and unevenly. In a Giemsa-stained preparation, the capsule surrounding *C. neoformans* can be seen as a clear unstained area. The histopathological examination of biopsy material can be done by staining with Mayer's mucicarmine (Colour plate VIII, Fig. 48), PAS, GMS and H & E staining.

Cultural characteristics

Sabouraud's dextrose agar

C. neoformans produces moist, white, cream coloured mucoid colonies usually after 2–3 days of incubation (Colour Plate VIII, Fig. 49). When examined microscopically, the yeast cells are capsulated but the capsules are often smaller than when seen in the specimens. Occasionally capsules are absent. Hyphae or pseudohyphae are not normally produced. *C. neoformans* is urease positive.

Niger seed agar/bird seed agar/caffeic acid agar

C. neoformans possesses the enzyme phenol oxidase, and testing for its presence is another means of accurate identification. *C. neoformans* produces black colonies on these media (Colour Plate VIII, Fig. 49).

Discussion

1. **Enumerate true yeasts.**
   - *Cryptococcus neoformans*
   - *Rhodotorula*
   - *Saccharomyces cerevisae*
2. **What are yeasts?**
   Yeasts are round, oval or elongated unicellular fungi which reproduce by simple budding.
3. **Name the reservoir of *C. neoformans*.**
   Pigeon droppings provide a reservior of the organisms.
4. **Name one staining technique to demonstrate *C. neoformans* capsule in biopsy materials.**
   Mayer's mucicarmine stain
5. **Enumerate the lesions produced by *C. neoformans*.**
   - Pulmonary lesions
   - Meningitis

Practical 44

Aspergillus

Introduction

Aspergillus species are saprophytic molds. *Aspergillus fumigatus* is the commonest human pathogen. Other species causing infection include *A. niger, A. flavus, A. terreus* and *A. nidulans.* Aspergillosis is caused by inhalation of *Aspergillus* conidia or mycelial fragments which are present on vegetation, decaying matter, soil and air.

Direct microscopy

Ten per cent KOH preparation

KOH preparation of sputum, bronchoalveolar lavage and other specimens reveal non-pigmented septate hyphae, 3–5 µm in diameter with characteristic dichotomous branching. The hyphae have a tendency to branch repeatedly. The branches arise at an angle of approximately 45 degrees. In a majority of lesions, only hyphal forms are seen.

Histological sections

It can be stained with H&E and GMS stains and examined for characteristic hyphae (Colour Plate VIII, Fig. 50).

Cultural characteristics

SDA

Colonies on SDA appear after incubation for 1–2 days at 25°C. The isolate is identified on the basis of growth characteristics and microscopic morphology. LCB mount shows branching and septate hyphae. From the latter arise condiophores, the ends of which are expanded to form vesicles. The vesicle bears one or two layers of sterigmata (phialides) which in turn bear conidia (Fig. 44.1).

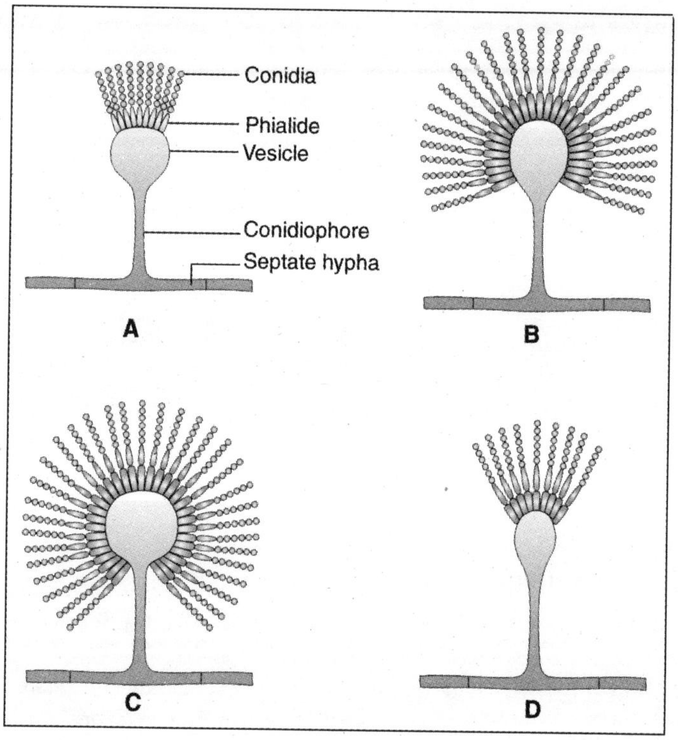

Fig. 44 .1. *Aspergillus* spp. : (A) *A. fumigatus,* (B) *A. flavus,* (C) *A. niger,* and (D) *A. terreus.*

Discussion

1. **Which species of *Aspergillus* is the commonest human pathogen?**
   A. fumigatus

2. **Enumerate the lesions produced by *Aspergillus.***
   - Allergic bronchopulmonary aspergillosis
   - Intracavitary aspergilloma (fungus ball)

- Invasive aspergillosis
- Endocarditis
- Paranasal granuloma

3. **Which SDA medium is used for growth of *Aspergillus*?**

   SDA without cycloheximide is used and incubated at 25°C.

4. **Name toxin produced by *Aspergillus.***

   Aflatoxin

5. **What do you mean by term 'uniseriate' and 'biseriate'?**

   Uniseriate **:** The vesicle is covered with only a single row of sterigmata.

   Biseriate **:** The vesicle is covered with two rows of sterigmata.

6. **Enumerate characteristic features of *Aspergillus* hyphae.**
   - Hyphae are non-pigmented.
   - They are septate, 3–5 µm in diameter with characteristic dichotomous branching.
   - The branches arise at an angle of approximately 45 degrees.

Practical 45

Zygomycetes

Introduction

Zygomycois or mucormycosis is an opportunistic infection caused by saprophytic fungi, notably species of *Mucor, Rhizopus* and *Absidia* of the family Mucoraceae. These fungi are common saprophytes of soil, manure and decaying vegetables, and fruits. These are essentially opportunistic fungi. The major predisposing factors to zygomycosis are diabetes mellitus, leukaemia or lymphoma and immunosuppression. The characteristic pathological changes in zygomycosis are suppuration and necrosis. Invasion of thrombosed blood vessels by the fungus is a conspicuous feature.

Direct microscopy

KOH preparation

KOH preparation of scrapings from the lesions, pus, sputum and nasal discharge shows irregularly branched, non-septate, thin-walled very broad hyphae (7–15 μm in diameter). True septa are rarely seen in the hyphae but under low magnification, cross folds in the walls of the hyphae may resemble septa.

Histological sections

The fungi are deeply stained with routine H & E stain. On

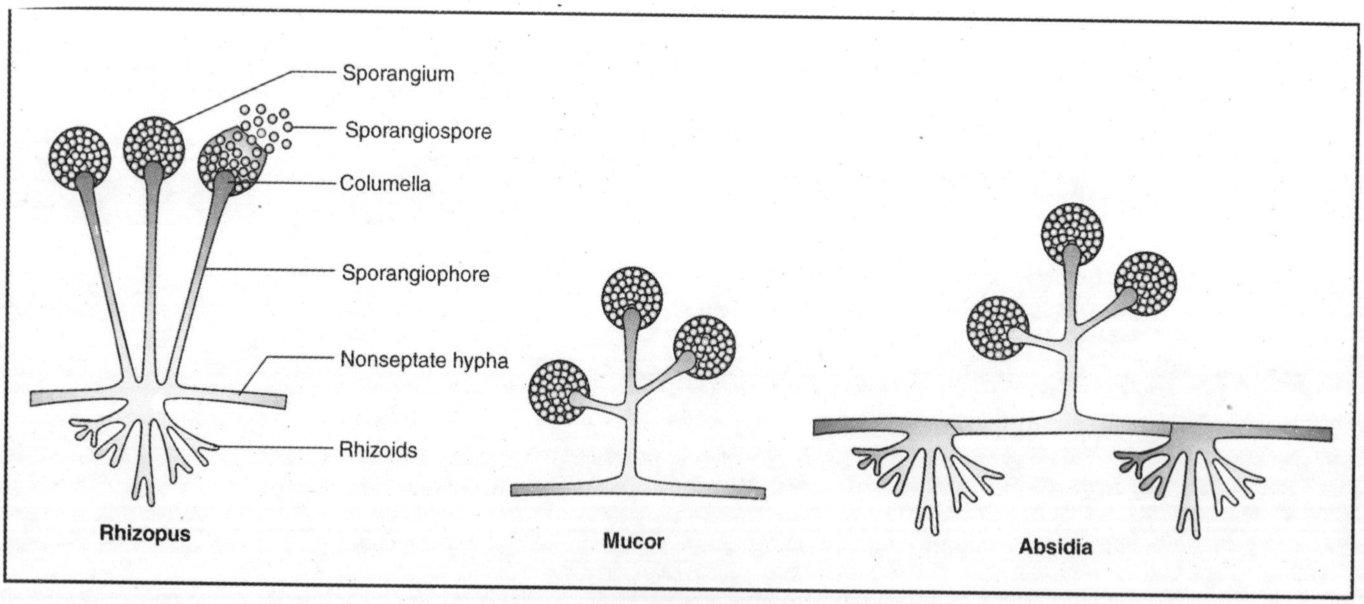

Fig. 45.1. *Rhizopus, Mucor and Absidia.*

the other hand, colouration by special fungal stain such as Gridley, PAS and in some cases GMS may be very poor.

Cultural characteristics

Fungi can be readily isolated on SDA at 37°C. *Rhizopus* has rhizoids and sporangiophores that arise in groups directly above the rhizoids. *Mucor* does not possess rhizoids and shows branched sporangiophores arising randomly along aerial mycelium. *Absidia* has rhizoids and sporangiophores that arise from the aerial mycelium in between the rhizoids (Fig. 45.1).

Discussion

1. **Name fungi which can invade blood vessels.**
   - *Aspergillus*
   - *Mucor*
   - *Rhizopus*
   - *Absidia*
2. **Enumerate pathogenic lesions produced by fungi of the class Zygomycetes.**
   - Rhinocerebral zygomycosis
   - Pulmonary zygomycosis
   - Gastrointestinal zygomycosis
   - Disseminated zygomycosis
   - Dermal zygomycosis
   - Subcutaneous zygomycosis
3. **Enumerate predisposing factors to mucormycosis.**
   - Diabetes mellitus
   - Metabolic acidosis
   - Leukaemia
   - Lymphoma
   - Immunosuppression
   - Widespread use of broad spectrum antibiotics, steroids and antimetabolites
4. **Which fungus does not possess rhizoids?**

   Mucor
5. **Describe the characteristic features of hyphae of Zygomycetes.**

   Hyphae are large ribbon-like irregularly branched, non-septate, broad and thin-walled. Hyphae may appear folded, twisted and distorted.

Practical 46

Dermatophytes

Introduction

Dermatophytes infect keratinized tissues of the skin, hair and nails. Dermatophytosis, tinea or ringworm is the most common type of superficial mycosis seen in human beings. Dermatophytosis is caused by 42 species of dermatophytes which belong to three genera (*Trichophyton, Microsporum* and *Epidermophyton*). On the basis of their natural habitat and host preferences, they are classified into three groups: geophilic, zoophilic and anthropophilic species.

Direct microscopy

KOH preparation

KOH preparation of skin scrapings, hair and nail clippings reveals branching septate hyphae or chains of arthroconidia. Three types of hair infection may be distinguished in wet mounts: ectothrix, endothrix and favic-type hair invasion.

Ectothrix : In this, the hyphae are sparsely distributed within hair shaft with a sheath of arthrospores on the surface of hair shaft. It is caused by *M. audouinii, M. canis* and *T. mentagrophytes* (Fig. 46.1A).

Endothrix : In this, the arthrospore formation occurs entirely within the hair completely filling the hair shaft. This is caused by *T. tonsurans* and *T. violaceum* (Fig. 46.1B).

Favus : In this, there is sparse hyphal growth and formation of air spaces within the hair shaft. This is caused by *T. schoenleinii* (Fig. 46.1C).

Demonstration of fungus in nails may be possible only after clearing with KOH for a day or two.

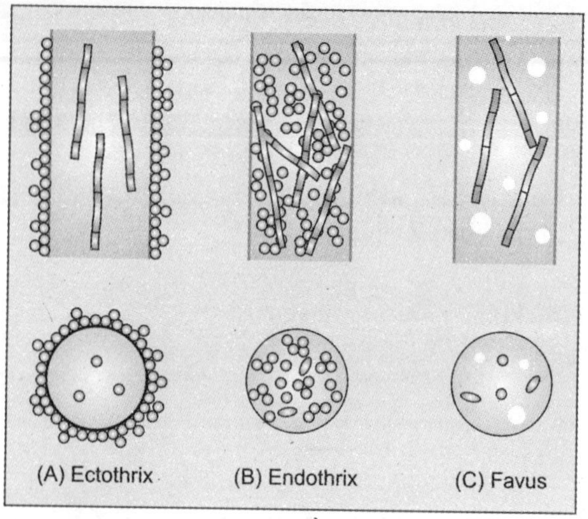

Fig. 46.1. Hair invasion of dermatophytes in longitudinal and transverse sections : (A) ectothrix, (B) endothrix, and (C) favus.

Culture

Species identification is possible only by culture examination. Keratinous material is inoculated on SDA with chloramphenicol and cycloheximide and incubated at 27–30°C for three weeks. Identification of dermatophytes is based on colonial morphology, colour, pigment production and production of microconidia and macroconidia (Fig. 46.2).

Trichophyton

Colonies may be powdery, velvety or waxy with pigmentation characteristic of different species. Macroconidia are usually rare but microconidia are abundant. The latter are

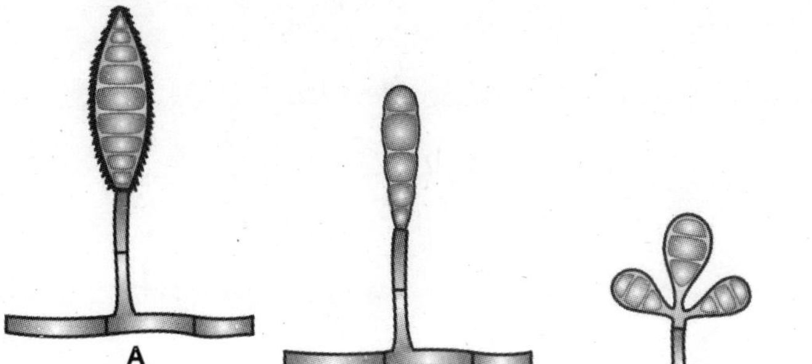

Fig. 46.2. Macroconidia in the three genera of dermatophytes : (A) *Microsporum*, (B) *Trichophyton*, and (C) *Epidermophyton.*

arranged in clusters along the hyphae or borne on conidiophores. Fungi of this genus can infect skin, hair and nails.

Microsporum

Colonies of the fungi of this genus are cottony, velvety or powdery with white to brown pigmentation. Macroconidia are very numerous and microconidia are relatively scanty. They infect skin and hair but not the nails.

Epidermophyton

Colonies are powdery and greenish-yellow. Microconidia are absent and macroconidia are club-shaped and are arranged in groups of two or three. It infects skin and nails but not hair.

Discussion

1. **Define dermatophytosis.**

   Dermatophytosis is superficial mycosis seen in human beings. It infects keratinized tissues of the skin, hair and nails.

2. **Define dermatomycosis.**

   The infection of skin caused by non-dermatophytic fungi and the cutaneous manifestations of systemic mycoses are known as dermatomycosis.

3. **Enumerate three genera of dermatophytes.**
   - *Trichophyton*
   - *Microsporum*
   - *Epidermophyton*

4. **Which factor is considered to differentiate three genera of dermatophytes?**

   The differentiation of the three genera is based mainly on the nature of macrocondia.

5. **In which genus macroconidia are usually rare?**

   In *Trichophyton* macroconidia are usually rare.

6. **Club-shaped macroconidia are present in which genus of dermatophytes?**

   Club-shaped macroconidia are present in *Epidermophyton.* They are arranged in groups of two or three.

7. **Define dermatophytid or id reaction.**

   Hypersensitivity to fungal antigens may lead to secondary eruptions occurring in sensitized patients because of circulation of allergenic products from the primary site of infection. It is known as dermatophytid or id reaction.

PART–6

Virology

Contents

Practical 47

Diagnostic Approach to Viral Infections

Specimen collection

Specimen for diagnosis of viral infections include: throat swab, nasopharyngeal swab, bronchial lavage, blood, bone marrow, rectal swab, stool, urine, sterile body fluids, tissues, skin smears, CSF and serum. Specimen should be collected as early as possible following the onset of infection.

Specimen transport

Viral transport media are used to transport swabs, tissues, scrapings or fluid specimens. Transport media contain protein, such as serum, albumin or gelatin and antimicrobials to prevent contamination by bacteria and fungi. Following transport media are used:

- Hanks balanced salt solution
- Eagles tissue culture medium
- Leibovitz-Emory medium

Specimen processing

All specimens for isolation of virus should be processed immediately. In case of delay, specimens should be stored in viral transport medium at 4°C. Processing should be done in a biological safety cabinet. Prior to processing requisition form should be seen for following information: date and time of specimen collection, source of specimen, clinical history and suspected viruses. Laboratory diagnosis of viral infections can be carried out by the following methods:

- Direct detection of virus, viral antigen or viral genome
- Virus isolation
- Detection of specific antiviral antibodies
- Cytological or histological examination of cells from the site of infection

Direct detection of virus, viral antigen or viral genome

Electron microscopy (EM)

Electron microscopy is one of the most useful tools for the direct demonstration of viruses in patients. On the basis of their distinctive appearances, most of the viruses can be assigned to the correct family. Viruses that are difficult to culture (rotavirus, astroviruses) can be recognized by electron microscopy. The clinical material can be negatively stained with potassium phosphotungstate or uranyl acetate and scanned by EM. Clinical applications of electron microscopy include detection of rotavirus and hepatitis A virus in faecal specimens, poxviruses in vesicle fluid and herpesvirus in brain biopsy tissue.

Immunoelectron microscopy

EM as a diagnostic tool has low sensitivity. For satisfactory results, the specimen should contain 10^7 virions per ml. The sensitivity of electron microscopy can be increased by mixing specific antibody with the specimen to aggregate the virus particles. These aggregates can be sedimented, centrifuged, negatively stained and observed under EM.

Fluorescence microscopy

Virions or viral antigens can be detected in frozen tissue sections, acetone-fixed cell smears, cells from virus infected cultures or vesicle fluid by direct or indirect fluorescent antibody technique. Fluorescence microscopy of brain biopsy can be used for the diagnosis of herpes simplex encephalitis and subacute sclerosing panencephalitis (a late sequelae of measles) and for the verification of rabies in the brain of animals suspected to be rabid. This method is also useful for the rapid diagnosis of respiratory infections caused by paramyxoviruses, orthomyxoviruses, adenoviruses and herpesviruses.

Light microscopy

Viral antigens in infected cells can be detected by immunoperoxidase staining. Tissue section or smear of infected cells is stained with antibody coupled to horseradish peroxidase. Hydrogen peroxide together with a benzidine derivative is then added. It forms a coloured insoluble precipitate which can be seen under ordinary light microscope.

Serological tests

Viral antigens may be detected by direct and indirect ELISA, radioimmunoassay and latex agglutination.

Nucleic acid probes

Enzyme-labelled or radiolabelled nucleic acid (DNA or RNA) sequences complementary to unique regions in nucleic acid sequences of most viruses are now manufactured commercially. These labelled complementary sequences are known as nucleic acid probes. Two strands of the target DNA molecule in the clinical specimens are first separated by boiling, then, following cooling, allowed to hybridize with a labelled single-stranded DNA or RNA probe present in excess. Depending on the type of label attached to the probe, hybridized-labelled probe can be detected by radiography, gamma-counting or a simple colourimetric evaluation (dot-blot hybridization). By use of nucleic acid probes cytomegalovirus, papillomavirus and Epstein-Barr virus have been identified. In situ hybridization may be used to detect integrated or nonintegrated copies of viral genome in persistent infections or viral cancers. Southern blot hybridization and Northern blot hybridization can be used for detection of DNA and RNA respectively.

Polymerase chain reaction (PCR)

It is a DNA amplification system that allows molecular biologists to produce microgram quantities of DNA from picogram amounts of starting material. It is based on repeated cycles of high temperature template denaturation, oligonucleotide primer annealing and polymerase mediated extension. With the revolutionary PCR technique, a target DNA sequence can be amplified at least 100,000 folds in just a few hours, a sharp contrast to the days required for conventional amplification method (culture). Thus viral DNA extracted from a very small number of virions or infected cells can be amplified to the point where it can readily be identified using labelled probes in a hybridization assay. For the detection of viral RNA, it is first converted into DNA by reverse transcriptase. PCR can be used for diagnosis of infections caused by HIV-1, HIV-2, HTLV-1, cytomegalovirus, human papillomavirus, herpes simplex viruses, HBV, HCV, HDV, HEV, rubella virus, Epstein-Barr virus, varicella-zoster virus, human herpes virus 6 and 7, parvovirus B19, enteroviruses, coxsackieviruses, echoviruses, rhinoviruses, measles virus and rotavirus.

Virus isolation

Most of the viruses can be cultivated in laboratory animals, chick embryos and cell cultures. Laboratory animals have now almost disappeared from virus diagnostic laboratories, because simpler methods such as cell cultures are available. Embryonated eggs offer several sites for the cultivation of viruses. Chorioallantoic membrane (CAM), allantoic cavity, amniotic cavity and yolk sac (Fig. 47.1) of 8–11 days old eggs are inoculated and incubated for 2–9 days. The duration of incubation depends on the virus type and route of inoculation. Viruses may kill the embryo or may produce visible lesions like pocks and haemagglutinating activity in the harvested amniotic and allantoic fluid. These effects help in the identification of the virus. Many viruses can be grown in eggs (Table 47.1), but it is now rarely used other than for the demonstration

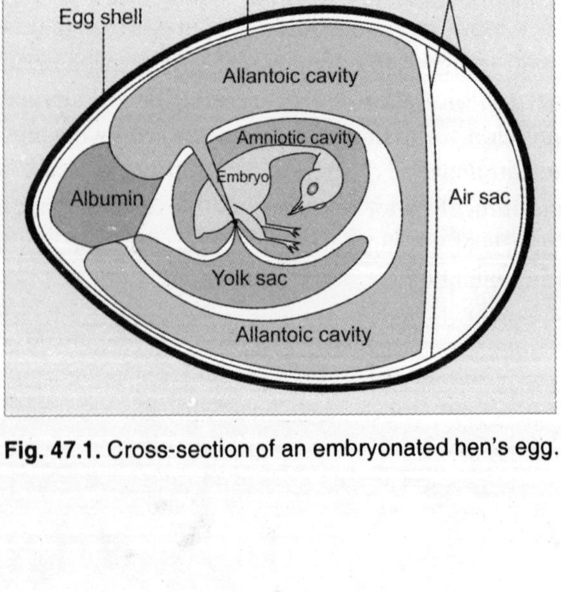

Fig. 47.1. Cross-section of an embryonated hen's egg.

Table 47.1. Virus isolation in chick embryo

Route of inoculation	*Virus*	*Demonstration of virus*			
		Lesion on CAM	*Haemaggluti-nation*	*Usually also kill the embryo*	*Rapidly lethal for embryo*
CAM	Poxviruses	+	–	–	–
	Herpes simplex	+	–	–	–
	Herpes B virus	+	–	–	–
Amniotic cavity	Influenza	–	+	–	–
	Mumps	–	+	–	–
Allantoic cavity	Newcastle disease	–	+	–	–
	Sendai	–	+	–	–
Yolk sac or CAM	Japanese B encephalitis	+	–	+	–
	St. Louis encephalitis	+	–	+	–
	West Nile virus	+	–	+	–
Any route	Equine encephalitis viruses	–	–	–	+

of poxviruses and the propagation of orthomyxoviruses and paramyxoviruses.

Cell culture

This is the type of culture routinely employed for diagnostic virology and for studying virus-cell interactions. Cell culture is of three types:

- *Primary cell culture*
- *Semi-continuous (diploid) cell culture*
- *Continuous cell lines*

Detection of virus growth in cell culture

Virus growth in cell culture can be detected by the following methods:

1. Cytopathic effect (CPE)

Many viruses produce morphological changes in the cultured cells in which they grow. These changes are known as cytopathic effects (CPE) and viruses causing CPE are known as cytopathogenic viruses. Most CPE can be readily observed in unfixed and unstained monolayer of cells under low power of microscope. But fixation and staining of monolayer is essential in order to see details such as inclusion bodies and syncytia. Conventional haematoxylin and eosin is most suitable for this purpose. Fluorescent antibody staining is widely used to recognize viral antigens in such cultured cells. Following are the main types of CPE:

Rounding of cells : Viral replication may lead to nuclear pyknosis, rounding, refractility, degeneration and eventually complete or partial detachment of infected cells from the glass. This is seen in picornaviruses.

Rounding and aggregation : Some viruses may lead to cell rounding and aggregation into grape-like clusters which detach from the glass, leaving clear areas. It is seen in adenoviruses.

Syncytium formation : Some viruses (measles, respiratory syncytial virus, HIV) lead to syncytium formation in which infected cells fuse with neighbouring infected or uninfected cells to form giant cells containing several (up to 100) nuclei.

Inclusion bodies : These are intranuclear or cytoplasmic aggregates of products of viral replication such as virus particles ready for release, over-production of a particular viral protein or proteins or some aberrant cellular structure such as clumped chromatin. They can be seen in stained preparation under a light microscope. They may be present in the cytoplasm or in the nucleus, or both of infected cells and may be acidophilic or basophilic, single or multiple, large or small and round or irregular (Fig. 47.2). Vaccinia and rabies viruses produce intracytoplasmic inclusion bodies, and adenoviruses and herpesviruses produce intranuclear inclusions. Inclusion bodies of measles virus are seen in both the locations.

2. Haemadsorption

Some orthomyxoviruses (influenza) and paramyxoviruses (parainfluenza, measles and mumps) code for red cell agglutinins which are incorporated into the cell membrane during infection, so that erythrocytes adhere to the infected cells. This adherence of erythrocytes to the infected cells is known as haemadsorption. It can be used to recognize infection with non-cytocidal viruses, as well as the early

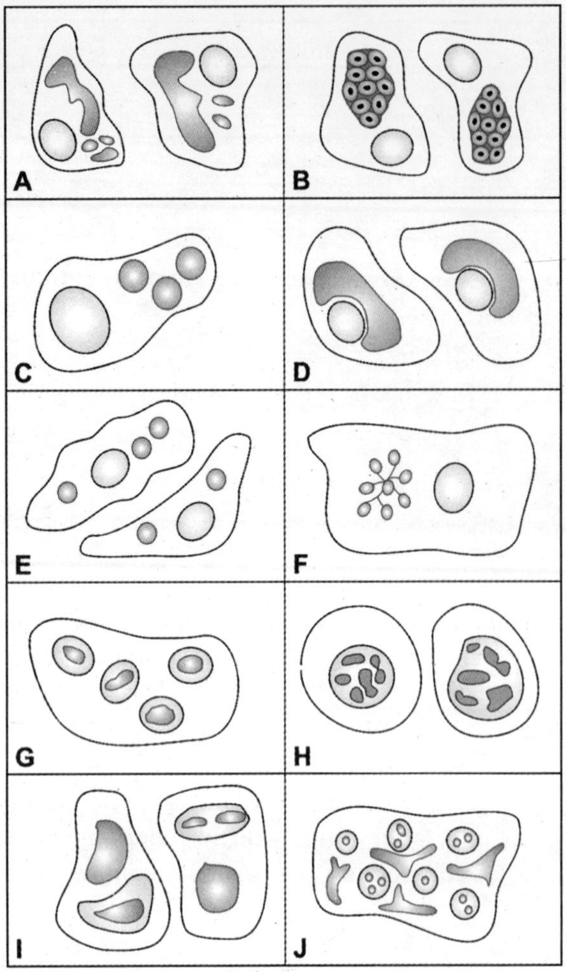

Fig. 47.2. Inclusion bodies in virus-infected cells. Intracytoplasmic (A–F) : A, Vaccinia virus (Guarnieri bodies); B, Molluscipox virus (Molluscum body); C, Fowlpox virus (Bollinger bodies); D, Reovirus; E, Rabies virus (Negri bodies); F, Respiratory syncytial virus. Intranucear (G–H) : G, Herpes simplex virus; H, Adenovirus. Intracytoplasmic and intranuclear both (I–J) : I, Cytomegalovirus; J, Measles virus.

stage of cytocidal viruses. Sometimes viruses can be detected by haemagglutination in the medium (culture fluid).

3. Interference

The multiplication of one virus in a cell usually inhibits the multiplication of a second virus, called the challenge virus, when it is added to the culture. This is because the first virus interferes with the replicative process of the challenge virus and is known as interference challenge test. This can be used for the detection of the growth of a non-cytopathogenic virus in cell culture. A cell culture is inoculated with suspected clinical sample and incubated for several days. Then a standard dose of a known cytopathogenic challenge virus is introduced into the culture and after incubation, culture is observed for the CPE of challenge virus. If virus from original inoculum was replicating within the cells, replication of the challenge virus will be prevented and no CPE will be seen in the culture.

4. Transformation

Tumour-forming (oncogenic) viruses induce cell transformation and loss of normal contact inhibition, so that growth appears in a piled-up fashion producing microtumours. Some herpesviruses, adenoviruses, hepadnaviruses, papovaviruses and retroviruses (human T cell lymphotropic virus type 1) can transform cells.

5. Fluorescent antibody testing

Cells from virus infected cultures can be stained with fluorescein-conjugated antiserum and seen under fluorescence microscope for virus antigens. Both direct (DFA) and indirect fluorescent antibody (IFA) methods are useful in the identification of viral culture isolates. DFA testing is the most convenient method for identifying many viral isolates. It provides a complete identification in less than one hour.

6. Immunoperoxidase staining

Direct immunoperoxidase (DIP) staining method may also be used in identification of viruses isolated in cell culture.

7. Detection of enzymes

The virus isolate can be identified by detection of viral enzymes, such as reverse transcriptase in retroviruses, in the culture fluid.

8. Electron microscopy

Viruses have distinctive appearances and can be detected by electron microscopy of ultra thin sections of infected cells.

Detection of specific antiviral antibodies

Using panels of known antigens, a number of serological techniques may be used to detect specific viral antibodies. Paired sera should be collected from the patient, the 'acute-phase' serum sample collected as early as possible in the illness and the 'convalescent-phase' sample collected at least 2 weeks later. Antibodies in the serum samples can be detected by ELISA, RIA, Western blot, latex agglutination, virus neutralization, haemagglutination inhibition, immunoflourescence, immunodiffusion and complement fixation tests.

Cytological or histologial examination of cells from the site of infection

Virus-induced histopathology (multinucleate giant cells and inclusion bodies) may be recognized by light microscopy.

Discussion

1. **Enumerate indications for laboratory diagnosis of viral infections.**
   - To detect emergence of drug-resistant mutants and for drug sensitivity testing.
   - To diagnose a disease for which antiviral chemotherapy is available.
   - Screening of blood donors for HIV, hepatitis B and C viruses.
   - Early detection of dangerous epidemics like yellow fever, poliomyelitis, encephalitis, etc.
   - For proper management of the patient.
2. **Enumerate viruses which can be detected in vesicular lesions of skin and mucous membrane.**
   - Herpes simplex
   - Varicella-zoster
   - Enteroviruses
3. **Enumerate viruses which cannot be cultivated in laboratory animals, chick embryo or cell cultures.**
   - Hepatitis B virus
   - Rotavirus
   - Papillomavirus
   - Some enteric viruses
4. **Enumerate various routes of inoculation in chick embryo.**
   - Chorioallantoic membrane (CAM)
   - Amniotic cavity
   - Yolk sac
5. **Enumerate viruses which can be propagated in amniotic cavity.**
   - Influenza
   - Mumps
6. **Classify various cell lines.**
   - Primary cell lines
   - Semi-continuous (diploid) cell lines
   - Continuous cell lines
7. **Enumerate various continuous cell lines.**
   - HeLa
   - HEp-2
   - KB
   - McCoy
   - Detroit 6
   - Vero
   - BHK-21
   - Chang C/I/L/K
8. **Enumerate viruses which show syncytium formation in cell culture.**
   - Measles
   - Respiratory syncytial virus
   - HIV
9. **Define inclusion bodies.**

   Inclusion bodies are intranuclear or cytoplasmic aggregates of products of viral replication such as viral particles, viral proteins or some aberrant cellular structure such as clumped chromatin.
10. **Enumerate viruses which produce intracytoplasmic inclusion bodies.**
    - Vaccinia virus
    - Rabies virus
11. **Name viruses which can be detected by electron microscopy.**
    - Rotatvirus
    - Hepatitis A virus
    - Poxviruses
    - Herpes viruses
12. **Enumerate various inclusion bodies seen in viral infections.**

Inclusion bodies	*Virus*
• Negri bodies	Rabies virus
• Guarnieri bodies	Vaccinia
• Bollinger bodies	Fowlpox
• Molluscum bodies	Molluscum contagiosum

13. **In which viral infection inclusions bodies are present in cytoplasm as well as nucleus?**

    Measles
14. **Enumerate oral manifestations of hepatitis C virus.**
    - Lichen planus
    - Oral malignancy
    - Salivary gland disease

15. **Where is the greatest concentration of HBV in the mouth?**
The greatest concentration of HBV is at the gingival sulcus.

16. **Enumerate hepatitis viruses which could be transmitted in dentistry.**
Hepatitis B, C, D and possibly hepatitis G

17. **Koplik's spots are characteristic of which viral disease?**
Measles

18. **What are the oral manifestations of herpes simplex virus?**
    - Cold sores of lips
    - Painful vesicles on the tongue and buccal mucosa

19. **Enumerate viral diseases causing lesions of the oral mucosa.**
    - Herpangina
    - Hand, foot and mouth disease
    - Warts
    - Herpes zoster
    - Infectious mononucleosis
    - Chickenpox
    - Recurrent herpes labialis
    - Recurrent intraoral herpes simplex
    - Primary acute herpetic gingivostomatitis
    - Primary HIV infection.

20. **What is the most common oral manifestation of HIV infection?**
Candidiasis

21. **Enumerate viruses causing lesions of oral mucosa in HIV infected patients.**
    - Herpes simplex virus
    - Varicella-zoster virus
    - Human papillomavirus
    - Cytomegalovirus
    - Epstein-Barr virus

PART–7

Recent Advances

Contents

Practical

48

Molecular Biology

Nucleic acid probes

Principle

The basic principle behind nucleic acid probe technology is hybridization of characterized nucleic acid probe to a specific nucleic acid sequence in a test specimen followed by detection of the paired hybrid. The hybridization reaction consists of four components :

- the probe,
- the target (which is contained in the sample),
- the reporter molecule, and
- the hybridization method.

Probe

A nucleic acid probe is a sequence of single-stranded nucleic acid that can hybridize specifically with its complementary strand via nucleic acid base pairing. A probe may be constructed to detect either DNA or RNA. All microorganisms, simple or complex, contain some unique sequences of DNA or RNA within their genome that distinguish them from all other organisms. The method of developing a nucleic acid probe (either DNA or RNA) is to cut or isolate those sequences from the nucleic acid of the cell using a set of enzymes known as restriction endonucleases, reproduce them in large quantities and attach a reporter molecule to them so that they can be incorporated into a hybridization process. The probe may be synthetically produced from oligonucleotide of specific sequences.

Target

The nucleic acid in the sample is referred to as the target. The sample may be a suspension of an unknown organism (for culture confirmation) or a clinical specimen such as sputum or stool.

Reporter molecule

The label on the probe, whether it is a radioisotope or an enzyme, is referred to as the reporter molecule. It helps to detect the hybridization reaction that may have occurred between probe and target. These include:

- Radioactive labels
  - ^{32}P
  - ^{125}I
  - ^{35}S
- Digoxigenin
- Chemiluminescense label
- Biotin-avidin
- Enzymes
  - Alkaline phosphatase
  - Horseradish peroxidase

Hybridization

This is the process whereby two single strands of nucleic acid come together to form a stable double-stranded molecule. However, they will bind and stay together only if the sequences of bases along each stretch of nucleic acid are complementary. Hybridization is accomplished in tubes or by spotting the unknown organisms on a filter paper such as nitrocellulose paper, lysing them to release DNA, and denaturing in mild alkali to single strands. The probe can then be added and after thorough washing to remove any unbound probe, the tube or probe is examined for evidence of hybridization. Depending upon the label (reporter molecule) hybridization can be detected by autoradiography, spectrophotometers or luminometers. Formalin-fixed, paraffin-embedded tissues can also be probed particularly for viral DNA sequences. DNA probes can also be designed that bind to RNA and this procedure has been used particularly to locate ribosomal RNA.

Applications of nucleic acid probes

- Rapid identification of organisms with long incubation time
- Direct detection of organisms in clinical specimens
- Confirmation of cultural isolates
- Detection of non-cultivable organisms
- Identification of toxins, virulence factors and resistance markers

Blotting

Blotting techniques are named according to the target molecule, which can be DNA, RNA and proteins.

Western blotting

In this technique, partially purified microbial preparation is first heated with a detergent such as sodium dodecyl sulphate (SDS). The SDS helps to release individual proteins from complex proteins. The proteins are separated according to their molecular weight on polyacrylamide gel by electrophoresis. The lower molecular weight proteins move readily through the gel matrix to the bottom of the gel. The separated proteins form invisible 'bands', in the gel. Now these separated protein bands on the surface of the gel are transferred to nitrocellulose membrane by blotting or electrophoresis. Nitrocellulose membrane is cut into strips after washing. A number of commercial kits for Western blotting contain nitrocellulose membrane strips on which the protein antigens of interest have been electrophoretically separated.

Test procedure

- The nitrocellulose membrane is immersed in diluted patient serum and incubated. Specific antibodies in the sample, if present, will bind to protein bands on the surface of nitrocellulose membrane during incubation.
- After incubation, the nitrocellulose membrane is thoroughly washed to remove unbound antibodies.
- After washing, the nitrocellulose membrane is incubated with enzyme tagged-antihuman gammaglobulin. Enzyme substrate is subsequently added which indicates positive test. The substrate changes colour in the presence of enzyme and permanently stains the nitrocellulose membrane. The position of the band on the membrane indicates the antigen (protein) with which the antibody has reacted.

Applications

- Supplemental test for HIV infection
- Diagnosis of Lyme disease
- Diagnosis of congenital syphilis

Southern blotting

DNA fragments obtained by restriction endonuclease enzyme are separated on the gel by electrophoresis. The separated DNA fragments are transferred to nitrocellulose membrane by blotting. The DNA bound to the membrane is denatured to single-stranded form and allowed to react with radioactive single-stranded DNA probes. Hybridization, if occurs, is further detected by autoradiography.

Northern blotting

In this technique, RNA mixture is separated by gel electrophoresis, blotted and probed with radioactive DNA or RNA.

Polymerase chain reaction (PCR)

Kary Mulis invented this method in 1989. He was awarded Nobel Prize in 1993. Polymerase chain reaction is a primer-mediated, temperature-dependent technique for the enzymatic amplification of a specific sequence (target sequence) to such an extent that it can be detected. The technique can be used to detect very small amount of specific nucleic acid material in clinical specimens where bacterial, viral, protozoal or fungal agents are thought to play a causative role. The fundamental basis of this technology is that each pathogenic organism possesses a unique 'signature sequence' in its DNA or RNA composition by which it can be identified. It is based on repeated cycles of high temperature template denaturation, oligonucleotide primer annealing, and polymerase mediated extension (Fig. 48.1).

To multiply a strip of genetic material, four ingredients are placed together in a small vial:

1. Target DNA.
2. Short strands of DNA called primers which tag the section to be copied.
3. Polymerase—an enzyme that promotes gene replication in all living cells.
4. Nucleotides—the building blocks for making DNA.

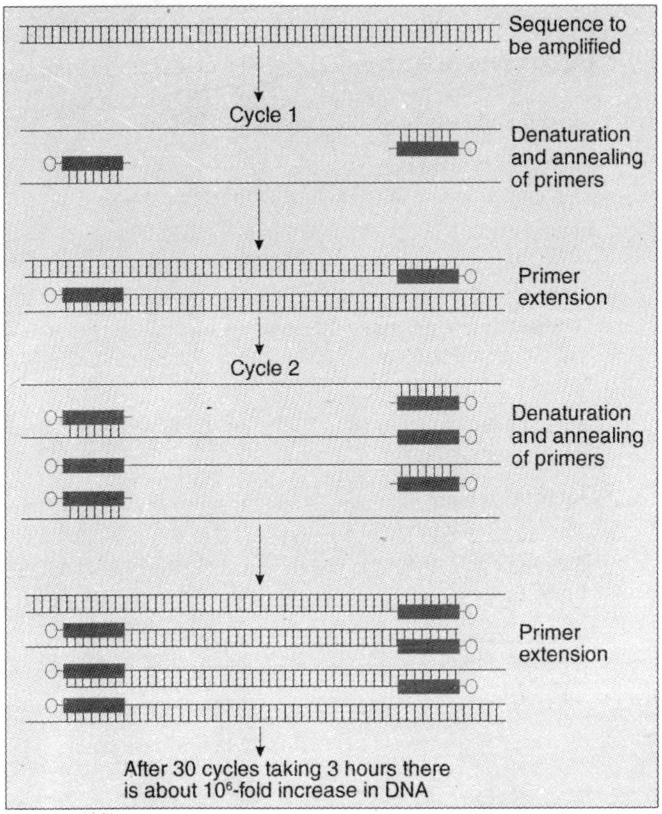

Fig. 48.1. Polymerase chain reaction.

PCR is carried out in three steps:

1. Heat at 94°C is applied to the target DNA, breaking the bonds that hold the strands together. This is known as **denaturation.**
2. The temperature is then reduced to 55°C, promoting the primers to attach themselves to either end of the target strip. This is known as **annealing** of primers.
3. Then polymerase enzyme triggers the formation of new DNA strand from the nucleotides. Extension of the primers is done by a thermostable *Taq* polymerase (purified from *Thermus aquaticus*, a thermophilic bacterium that lives in hot springs at temperature of 70–75°C). This is known as **primer extension**. When the temperature is again raised, the new strands separate and the process begins again.

These three steps are repeated again and again by manipulating the temperature, a process that is automated by the PCR machine (Table 48.1) A cycle takes about 3–5 minutes and after 30 cycles, taking about 2 hours, a single copy of DNA can be increased up to 1,000,000 copies, a sharp contrast to the days required by conventional amplification method (culture).

Table 48.1. Programming of cycles in polymerase chain reaction

Step	*Temperature*	*Time*	*Cycle*
Initial denaturation	94°C	5 minutes	First cycle
Denaturation	94°C	30 seconds	
Annealing of primers	55°C	1 minute	30 cycles
Primer extension	72°C	1 minute	
Final primer extension	72°C	7 minutes	Last cycle

Amplified sequences of target DNA can be detected by a variety of methods. If enough amplified DNA is present, it can be visualized by:

1. Gel electrophoresis and ethidium bromide staining.
2. Southern blot and dot-blot analysis with either radioactive or nonradioactive probes.
3. Oligomer restriction.
4. Oligomer hybridization.
5. Reverse dot-blot.

Reverse polymerase chain reaction

Instead of *Taq* polymerase described above, *Tth* polymerase obtained from *Thermus thermophilus* may be used. The *Tth* enzyme possesses both DNA polymerase and reverse transcriptase activities at high temperature. This allows both cDNA synthesis from mRNA followed by PCR amplification.

Applications of PCR

The development of PCR or gene amplification method is a major methodological breakthrough in molecular biology. Within a short span, this method has found its way into nearly every type of laboratory from forensic to ecology and from diagnosis to pure research.

Discussion

1. **Enumerate basic steps of nucleic acid probe technology.**
   - Preparation and labeling of single-stranded nucleic acid probe
   - Preparation of single-stranded target nucleic acid
   - Hybridization of target and probe nucleic acid
   - Detection of hybridization
2. **Enumerate viruses which can be detected directly in the specimens using probes.**
   - Enteroviruses

- Human papillomavirus
- Herpes simplex viruses

3. **Who discovered Southern blotting?**
   E. M. Southern

4. **What is the role of restriction endonuclease enzymes in molecular biology?**
   Restriction endonucleases cut double-stranded DNA at specific sequences and produce DNA fragments of varying length.

5. **Who invented polymerase chain reaction (PCR)?**
   Kary Mulis in 1989

6. **Enumerate three basic steps of a PCR cycle.**
   - Denaturation
   - Annealing
   - Primer extension

7. **How much time is taken in one cycle of PCR?**
   Three to five minutes

8. **Define polymerase chain reaction.**
   Polymerase chain reaction is a primer-mediated, temperature-dependent technique for the enzymatic amplification of a specific sequence to such an extent that it can be detected.

9. **At what temperature annealing of primers occur?**
   55°C

10. **In how many cycle of PCR, good amplification of DNA is obtained?**
    25–30 cycles

11. **How many copies of DNA are obtained at the end of PCR?**
    10^6 copies from a single copy of DNA

PART–8

Spots

Contents

Practical

49

Spots

1. McIntosh-Fildes' anaerobic jar

This is most reliable and widely used anaerobic jar. It is cylindrical vessel made of glass or metal with a metal lid, which is held firmly in place by a clamp. The lid has two tubes with taps, one acting as gas inlet and the other as the outlet (Fig. 49.1). On its undersurface, it carries a gauze sachet carrying alumina pellets coated with palladium. It acts as a room temperature catalyst for the conversion of hydrogen and oxygen into water. It acts as a catalyst, as long as the sachet is kept dry.

Inoculated culture plates are placed inside the jar and the lid is clamped tight. The outlet tube is connected to a vacuum pump and the air inside is evacuated. The outlet tap is then closed and the inlet tube connected to a hydrogen supply. Hydrogen is drawn in rapidly. As soon as this inrush of gas has ceased the inlet tap is also closed. After about 5 minutes inlet tap is again opened. There occurs again an immediate inrush of hydrogen since the catalyst creates a reduced pressure within the jar due to the conversion of hydrogen and leftover oxygen into water. The jar is left connected to hydrogen supply for about 5 minutes, then the inlet tap is closed and the jar is placed in the incubator, catalysis will continue until all the oxygen in the jar has been used up.

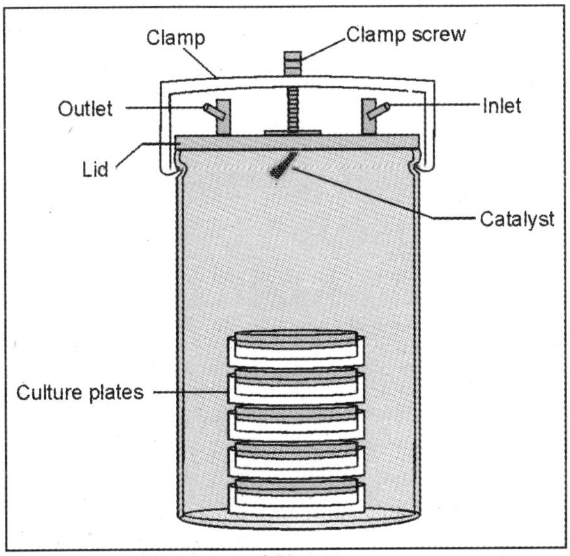

Fig. 49.1. McIntosh-Fildes' anaerobic jar.

Indicator

Methylene blue indicator is used for verifying the anaerobic condition in the jar. When it is placed in an anaerobic environment it is reduced from its coloured oxidized form to a colourless reduced leuco-compound. In place of chemical indicator, a culture plate inoculated with strict anaerobe such as *Clostridium tetani*, and a strict aerobe such as *Pseudomonas aeruginosa* may be used as biological indicator. Growth of strict anaerobe and no growth of strict aerobe indicates that anaerobiasis has been maintained.

2. GasPak envelope

The gasPak is now the method of choice for preparing anaerobic jar (Fig. 49.2). The gasPak is commercially available as a disposable envelope containing chemicals which generate hydrogen and carbon dioxide on the addition of water. After the inoculated plates are kept in the jar, the gasPak envelope with water added, is placed inside and lid is screwed tight. Hydrogen and carbon diox-

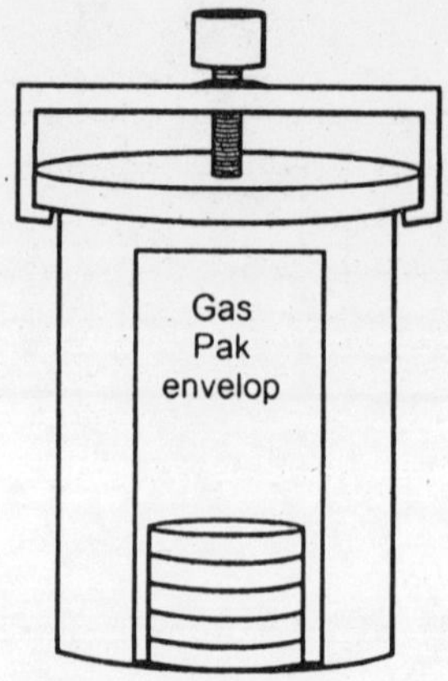

Fig. 49.2. GasPak anaerobic jar.

ide are liberated and the presence of a cold catalyst in the envelope permits the combination of hydrogen and oxygen to produce an anaerobic environment.

Advantages

- Operation of the jar is quick and simple.
- There is no need of vacuum pump and cylinder of compressed gas.

3. VDRL slide

It is a glass slide (7.5 × 5 cm) with 12 paraffin rings of approximately 15 mm diameter (Fig. 49.3). It is used to do VDRL test for diagnosis of syphilis. Slide tests require small quantities of antigen and antibody as compared to tube tests. Positive and negative reactions can be detected under microscope.

4. Seitz filter (Asbestos filter)

This is made up of a disc of asbestos (magnesium trisilicate). It is supported on a perforated metal disc within a metal funnel. The latter with filter disc is fitted on to a sterile flask through a silicone rubber bung (Fig. 49.4). The fluid to be sterilized is put into the funnel and the flask is connected to the exhaust pump through its side tap. Sterilized fluid is collected from the flask and filter disc is discarded after use. These discs are available with

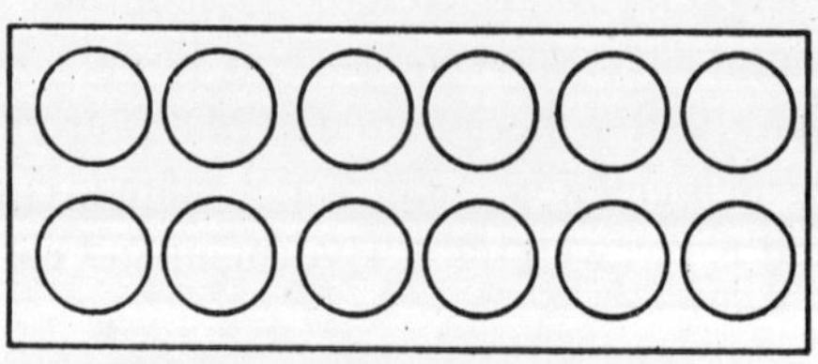

Fig. 49.3. VDRL slide.

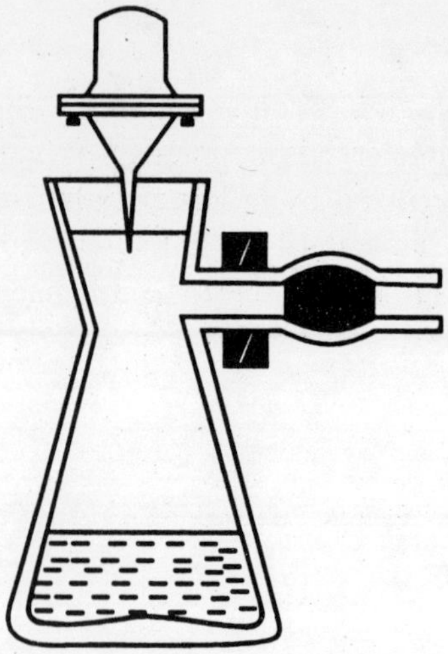

Fig. 49.4. Seitz filter.

different grades of porosity. *Serratia marcescens* and *Pseudomonas diminuta* have been used to test the efficacy of the filters.

Uses

- It is used to sterilize liquids such as sera and solutions of heat-labile substances such as sugars and urea, for preparation of media.
- It is also useful for separation of bacteriophages and bacterial toxins from bacteria and for the isolation of organisms which are scanty in fluids.

5. Swab stick

It is a thin wire or stick with cotton wrapped at one end. It is kept in a cotton plugged test tube (Fig. 49.5) and is sterilized in hot-air oven at 160°C for one hour or 180°C for 20 minutes.

Uses

- It is used for collection of clinical specimens like pus or other discharge.
- It is also used for preparing lawn culture on Mueller-Hinton agar to find out the antibiotic sensitivity pattern of bacteria.

Fig. 49.5. Swab stick.

6. Nichrome loop

The loop is flat, circular and completely closed with 2–4 mm internal diameter. It is mounted on a handle (Fig. 49.6). The loop is sterilized by holding it almost vertical in a bunsen burner flame until red hot. Owing to the high cost of platinum, loops for rountine work are made of nichrome, No. 24 SWG.

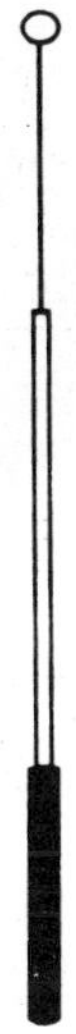

Fig. 49.6. Nichrome loop.

Uses

- It is used for inoculating various clinical specimens on solid or liquid media.
- It is used in streak culture and stroke culture.
- It is used to put up biochemical reactions.

7. Cavity slide

This is a glass slide with cavity. It is used to determine the motility of bacteria by hanging drop preparation. Some glass slides are available with twelve cavities and they are used to perform VDRL test for the diagnosis of syphilis.

8. Microtitre plate

It is a plastic plate with 96 wells (8 × 12) (Fig. 49.7). It is made up of polystyrene. It is used because small quantities of antigen and antibody required to conduct the test.

Uses

- It may be used to conduct ELISA test.
- It may be used to conduct Weil-Felix agglutination reaction and haemagglutination test.

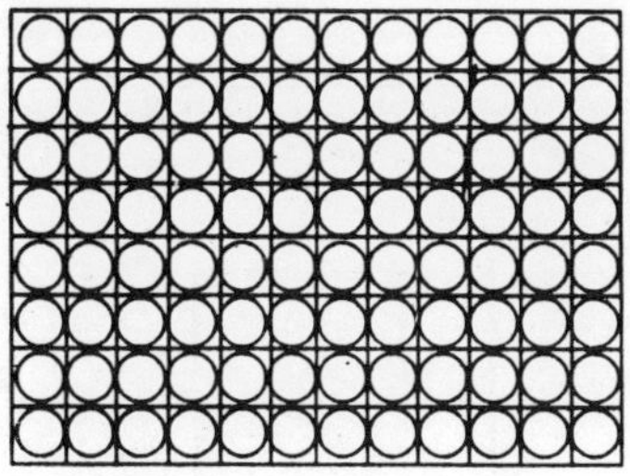

Fig. 49.7. Microtitre plate.

9. Antibiotic sensitivity plate

Kirby-Bauer disc diffusion method

The petri dish usually contains Mueller-Hinton agar. Inoculation is done on the dried surface of agar plate by streaking the swab three times over the entire agar surface. Antibiotic discs are placed on this plate. Usually not more than 7 discs are placed on one plate of 100 mm diameter. The plate is incubated at 35–37°C for 16–18 hours. Next day by using a transparent plastic ruler, the zones of complete growth inhibition around each of the discs are carefully measured (Fig. 14.1). The interpretation of zone size into susceptible, moderately susceptible or resistant is based on the interpretation chart.

10. Blood culture bottle

It is a glass bottle with a capacity of 150–200 ml. It contains metallic screw cap covered with sterilized paper (Fig. 49.8). It contains 50–100 ml volume of liquid culture medium (glucose broth, bile broth or brain-heart infusion broth). Five to 10 ml of blood is collected aseptically from antecubital vein and inoculated into blood culture bottle through a hole in screw cap. This is followed by incubation of bottle at 37°C. Depending upon the organisms sus-

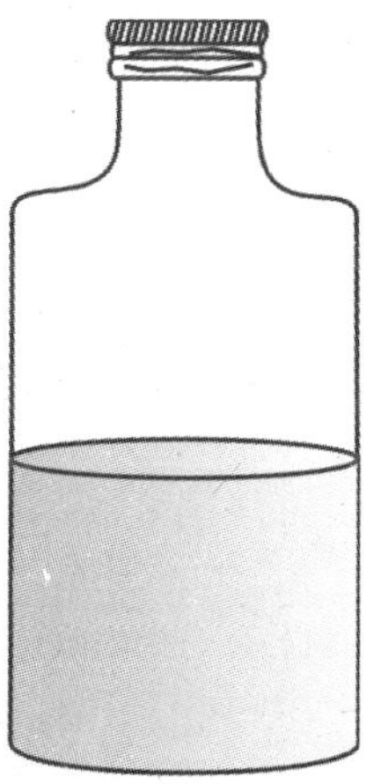

Fig. 49.8. Blood culture bottle.

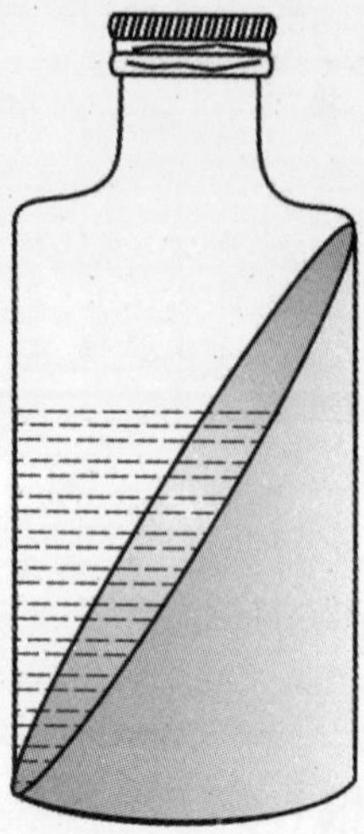

Fig. 49.9. Castaneda blood culture bottle.

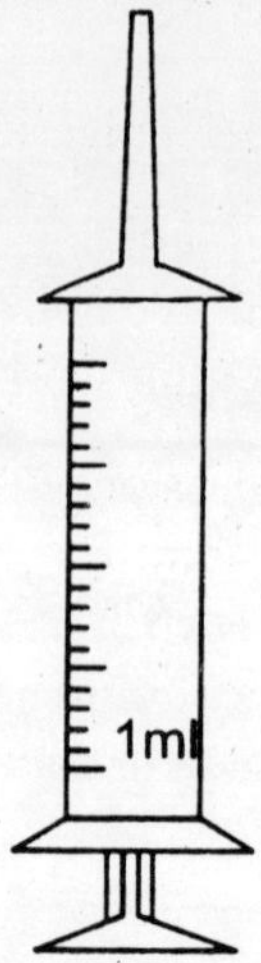

Fig. 49.10. Tuberculin syringe.

pected subcultures are made on appropriate culture plates at variable intervals. This method is useful to culture the blood of patients suffering from pyrexia of unknown origin and septicaemic patients.

11. Castaneda blood culture medium

This blood culture bottle contains both liquid serum dextrose broth and solid serum dextrose agar media (Fig. 49.9). Five to 10 ml of blood, collected aseptically from antecubital vein, is inoculated into the broth and bottle incubated in the upright position. For subculture, the bottle is tilted so that the broth flows over the surface of agar slant. It is again incubated in upright position. In positive cases, colonies appear on the slant. This is most definitive method for the diagnosis of brucellosis.

Advantages

This technique reduces the chances of contamination and risk of infection to laboratory personnel.

12. Tuberculin syringe

It is 1 ml glass syringe. Sterilized plastic syringes are also available (Fig. 49.10).

Uses

- It is used to conduct Mantoux test.
- It can be used to inject insulin.
- It can be used to inject antigen to conduct various skin hypersensitivity tests.
- It can be used to inject small amount of test material into animal.

13. Glass syringes

Glass syringes are available in different capacities and these are sterilized in hot air oven at 160ºC for 1 hour or 180ºC for 20 minutes.

Uses

- These are used to withdraw blood or fluids from patients for conducting diagnostic tests.
- These are also used to withdraw blood from animals to prepare blood agar plate.
- These are used to give intramuscular or intravenous injections to patients.

14. Plastic syringes

Sterilized disposable plastic syringes are also available. These are sterilized by gamma radiations and ethylene oxide. This method of sterilization is known as **cold sterilization**. They can be used for all those procedures where we use glass syringes.

15. Disinfectants

Disinfectants are antimicrobial agents used to kill potentially infectious agents present on inanimate objects. Antiseptics (mild disinfectant) are non-toxic antimicrobial agents that may be applied topically to the body surface either to kill or inhibit the growth of pathogenic organisms. The disinfectant may be dispensed in bottle showing its identity. It may be phenol, cresol, dettol, glutaraldehyde, formalin, etc.

Uses

- Glutaraldehyde is used for sterilization of heat sensi-

tive instruments like cystoscopes, bronchoscopes, thermometers, etc.
- Formalin is used for fumigation of operation theatres, wards, laboratories, etc.
- Dettol may be used for cleaning wound.

16. Tissue culture bottle

It may be made up of glass or plastic (Fig. 49.11). It contains tissue culture medium. The medium is buffered with bicarbonate to give a pH of 7.2–7.4 and phenol red is added as a pH indicator. Antimicrobial agents are added to prevent bacterial and fungal contamination.

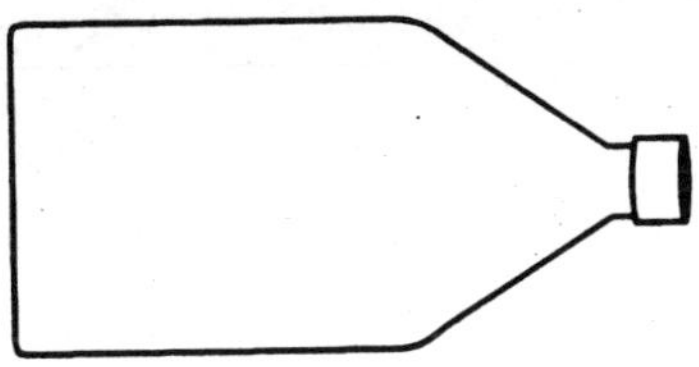

Fig. 49.11. Tissue culture bottle.

Uses

- They are used for propagation of cell lines.
- Cytopathic effect of viruses can be observed in the cultured cells.

17. Bijou bottle

It is a small screw-capped round glass bottle available in 15 ml capacity (Fig. 49.12).

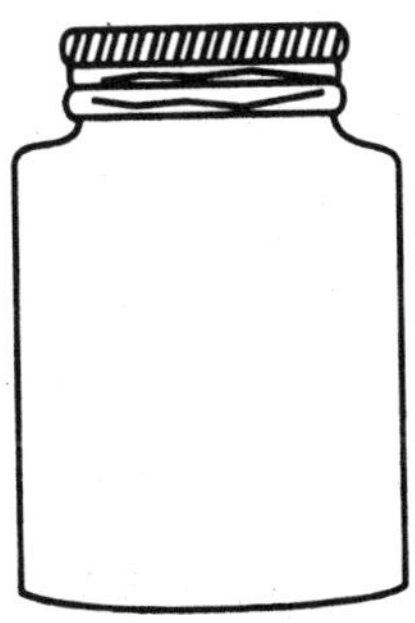

Fig. 49.12. Bijou bottle.

Uses

- It is used to maintain stock cultures of bacteria.
- It may be used for transportation of bacterial culture.

18. Dark-field condenser

Dark-field condenser is used for dark-field microscopy. By means of condenser the specimen is illuminated by oblique light only. The rays do not enter the tube of the microscope, and in consequence, do not reach the eye of the observer unless they are scattered by objects (e.g. bacteria) of different refractive index from the medium in which they are suspended. As a result, the organisms appear brightly illuminated against a dark background. It renders visible delicate organisms such as *Treponema pallidum*.

19. Petri dishes

Petri dishes of glass and plastic are routinely used in laboratory. After washing, glass petri dishes are sterilized in hot air oven at 160°C for one hour or 180°C for 20 minutes. The melted medium is poured in sterilized petri dishes and left undisturbed until the medium has set. Plastic petri dishes are available in two varieties i.e. disposable and reusable. Disposable are discarded after single use. Reusable are washed, sterilized by autoclaving and reused.

Uses

- They are used to prepare various solid culture media.
- They may be used for gross examination of stool sample.
- They are used to put up slide culture test for fungi.

20. Test tubes stoppered with cotton-wool plug

Test tubes of glass are routinely used in laboratory. They are available in different capacities. After washing and drying, they are stoppered with cotton plug and sterilized in hot air oven at 160°C for 1 hour or 180°C for 20 minutes. After each use they are discarded in jar containing disinfectant after removing the cotton plugs.

Uses

- They are used for pouring liquid media.
- They are used for preparation of solid media in the form of slopes e.g. Christensen medium and Simmon's citrate medium.
- They are used to put up biochemical reactions.

21. National institute of Health swab (NIH swab)

NIH swab consists of a glass rod at one end of which a piece of transparent cellophane (with sticky surface out) is wrapped and held in place with a rubber band. The other end of the glass rod is fixed in a rubber stopper and kept in a test tube (Fig. 49.13). The cellophane part is used for swabbing by rolling over the perianal and perineal area. Then the cellophane is detached, spread over glass slide

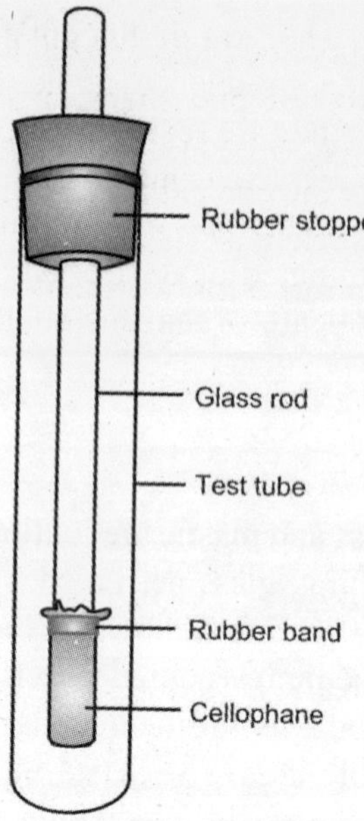

Fig. 49.13. NIH swab.

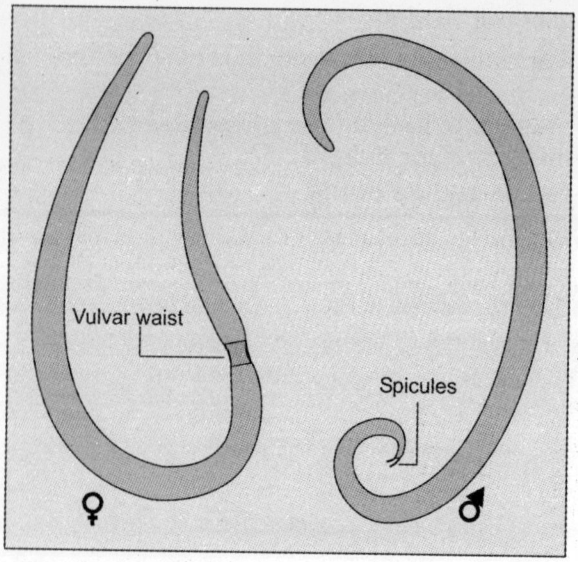

Fig. 49.14. Adult worms of *Ascaris lumbricoides.*

and examined microscopically. This procedure should be repeated on three successive days. Eggs of *Enterobius vermicularis* which are deposited in large numbers on the perianal and perineal skin at night can be demonstrated.

22. Ascaris lumbricoides (Round worm)

Adult worm

The body of *A. lumbricoides* is cylindrical tapering gradually at the anterior end and somewhat less so at the posterior end. White longitudinal streaks can usually be seen along the entire length of the pinkish cream body of the parasite (Fig. 49.14).

Male worm

It measures 15–30 cm in length and 3–4 mm in diameter. The posterior end is curved ventrally to form a hook. The ejaculatory duct along with the anus open into the cloaca from which arises a pair of copulatory spicules of equal size.

Female worm

It is longer and stouter than the male worm and measures 25–40 cm in length and 5 mm in diameter. The tail is straight and conical. The anus is subterminal and opens on the ventral surface in the form of a transverse slit. The vulva opens at the junction of the anterior and the middle thirds of the body on the midventral aspect of the worm. This part of the worm is narrower and is known as **vulvar waist.** A mature female lays nearly 200,000 eggs daily which are passed in the faeces.

23. Taenia saginata (The beef tapeworm; the unarmed tapeworm of man)

The adult worm consists of scolex (head), neck and strobila which is made up of a large number of proglottids (1,000–2,000). It is 4–6 metres or more in length. Scolex is large, quadrate without rostellum and hooklets, and possesses four suckers which may be pigmented.

Taenia solium (The pork tapeworm; the armed tapeworm of man)

It is 2–4 metres or more in length. Scolex is small, globular, with rostellum armed with a double row of 25–30 alternating large and small hooklets and possesses four suckers which are not pigmented. Number of proglottids is 800–1,000, which are expelled in chains of 5 or 6.

24. Hydatid cyst

It represents larval form of *Echinococcus granulosus* (Colour Plate VIII, Fig. 51). The cyst wall consists of ectocyst and endocyst. Ectocyst is outer layer. It is tough, acellular, laminated, hyaline membrane up to 1 mm in thickness. It is elastic, therefore, when excised or ruptured, it curls on itself thus exposing the inner layer containing brood capsules, scolices and daughter cysts. Endocyst is inner or germinal layer. It consists of a numher of nuclei embedded in a protoplasmic mass. It measures 22–25 μm in thickness. It gives rise to ectocyst on outside and brood capsules and scolices on inside (Colour Plate VIII, Fig.

52). It also secretes hydatid fluid. Hydatid fluid is clear, colourless or pale yellow with specific gravity 1.005–1.010. It is antigenic, therefore, it is used in Casoni test.

25. Fasciola hepatica (The sheep liver fluke; the common liver fluke)

It is a large leaf-shaped fluke measuring 30 mm × 13mm and brown to pale grey in colour. It is bilaterally symmetrical with three body layers, but has no true body cavity. At the anterior end there is distinct conical projection. The posterior end is broadly pointed. The oral sucker is situated in the conical projection at the anterior end. The ventral sucker is 1.6 mm in diameter and is situated nearby in a line with two shoulders.

PART–9

Appendices

Contents

APPENDIX-I

Notifiable Infectious Diseases

- Cholera
- Plague
- Anthrax
- Diphtheria
- Tetanus
- Leptospirosis
- Relapsing fever
- Typhus
- Meningococcal septicaemia
- Leprosy
- Tuberculosis
- Typhoid fever
- Malaria
- Smallpox
- Measles
- Mumps
- Rubella
- Rabies
- Acute poliomyelitis
- Viral haemorrhagic fever
- Acute encephalitis

Old nomenclature of few organisms

Old Nomenclature	*New Nomenclature*
• Klebs-Loeffler bacillus	*Corynebacterium diphtheriae*
• Preisz-Nocard bacillus	*Corynebacterium pseudotuberculosis*
• Friedlander's bacillus	*Klebsiella pneumoniae*
• Eberth-Gaffky bacillus or Eberthella typhi	*Salmonella* Typhi
• Whitmore's bacillus	*Burkholderia pseudomallei*
• Pfeiffer's bacillus	*Haemophilus influenzae*
• Koch-Weeks bacillus	*Haemophilus aegypticus*
• Bordet-Gengou bacillus	*Bordetella pertussis*
• Donovan's bacillus	*Calymmatobacterium granulomatis*
• Hansen bacillus	*Mycobacterium leprae*

APPENDIX-II

Characteristic colonial appearance

Appearance	***Organisms***
Oil-paint	*Staphylococcus aureus*
Draughtsman or carrom coin	*Streptococcus pneumoniae*
Daisy head	*Corynebacterium diphtheriae* biotype gravis
Frog's egg	*C. diphtheriae* biotype intermedius
Poached egg	*C. diphtheriae* biotype mitis
Medusa head	*Bacillus anthracis*
Bisected pearls or mercury drops	*Bordetella*
Aluminium paint (confluent growth)	*Bordetella*
Rough, tough and buff	*Mycobacterium tuberculosis*
Fried egg	*Mycoplasma*
Pitting or corroding	*Eikenella corrodens*
Molar tooth	*Actinomyces israelii*

Characteristic appearance of bacteria in stained-smear

Appearance	***Organisms***
Rail road track or school of fish	*Haemophilus aegypticus*
Thumb print	*Bordetella*
Fish in stream	*Vibrio cholerae*
Safety pin	*Yersinia pestis*
Drumstick	*Clostridium tetani*
Bamboo stick	*Bacillus anthracis*
Bunch of grapes	*Staphylococcus aureus*
Lanceolate or flame-shaped	*Streptococcus pneumoniae*
Kidney-shaped	*Neisseria gonorrhoeae* and *N. meningitidis*
Chinese letter arrangement	*Corynebacterium diphtheriae*
Cigar bundle	*Mycobacterium leprae*
Sun ray	*Actinomyces*

APPENDIX–III

Differentiation of organisms of family Enterobacteriaceae by biochemical tests

Biochemical tests	*Escherichia coli*	*Edwardsiella*	*Citrobacter freundii*	*Klebsiella pneumoniae*	*Enterobacter*	*Salmonella*	*Shigella*	*Hafnia*	*Serratia*	*Proteus*	*Provi–dencia*	*Morga–nella*	*Yersinia enteroco–litica*
Indole	+	+	–	–	–	–	v	–	–	v	+	+	v
MR	+	+	+	–	–	+	+	–	–	+	+	+	+
VP	–	–	–	+	+	–	–	+	+	–	–	–	v
Citrate	–	–	+	+	+	v	–	+	+	v	v	–	–
Urease	–	–	v	+	v	–	–	–	–	+	v	+	+
H_2S	–	+	+	–	–	+	–	–	–	+	–	–	–
Motility	+	+	+	–	+	+	–	+	+	+	+	+	+ at 22°C
Growth in KCN	–	–	+	+	+	–	–	+	+	+	+	+	–
PPA	–	–	–	–	–	–	–	–	–	+	+	+	–
Gelatin (22°C)	–	–	–	–	v	–	–	–	v	+	–	–	–
Malonate	–	–	v	+	v	–	–	v	–	–	–	–	–
Lysine decarboxylase	v	+	–	v	v	+	–	+	+	–	–	–	–
Arginine decarboxylase	v	–	v	–	v	+	–	v	–	–	–	–	–
Ornithine decarboxylase	v	+	v	–	+	+	v	+	+	v	–	+	+
ONPG	+	–	+	+	+	–	–	+	+	–	–	–	+
Acid from													
Glucose	+	+	+	+	+	+	v	+	v	+	v	+	–
Lactose	+	–	v	+	+	–	–	–	–	–	–	–	–
Sucrose	v	–	v	+	+	–	–	–	+	v	v	–	+
Mannitol	+	–	+	+	+	+	v	+	+	–	–	–	+

(v–variable)